FIRESIDE

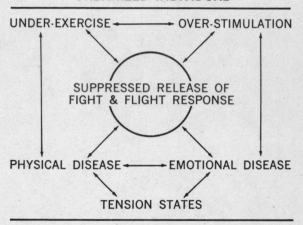

URBANIZED INDIVIDUAL

UNDER-EXERCISE ⟷ OVER-STIMULATION

SUPPRESSED RELEASE OF
FIGHT & FLIGHT RESPONSE

PHYSICAL DISEASE ⟷ EMOTIONAL DISEASE

TENSION STATES

BACKACHE

Stress and Tension

THEIR CAUSE, PREVENTION AND TREATMENT

HANS KRAUS, M.D.

A FIRESIDE BOOK
PUBLISHED BY SIMON AND SCHUSTER

Manufactured in the United States of America

1 2 3 4 5 6 7 8 9 10

Library of Congress Cataloging in Publication Data

Kraus, Hans, 1905-
    Backache stress and tension, their cause,
prevention and treatment.

    (A Fireside book)
    Bibliography: p.
    1.   Backache.   2.   Stress (Physiology)   3.   Ex-
ercise therapy.   I.   Title.   [DNLM: 1.   Backache—
Popular works.   2.   Stress—Popular works.
WE720 K91b   1965a]
RD768.K7   1978   617'.5   77-27374

    ISBN 0-671-06450-9
    ISBN 0-671-24214-8 Pbk.

For permission to use the following materials, the author wishes to thank:

Charles C Thomas—for material and illustrations from my books, *Principles and Practice of Therapeutic Exercises,* copyright © 1949, 1963, and *Hypokinetic Disease,* copyright © 1961.

The Lancet—for statistics from "Coronary Heart-disease and Physical Activity of Work," by Morris, J. N., Heady, J. A., Raffle, P. A., Roberts, C. G., and Parks, J. W., in *Lancet* 2:1053, November 21, 1953, and 2:1111, November 28, 1953.

Dr. Lloyd Appleton—for the graph on "Discharge of West Point Cadets with Psychiatric Endorsement."

New York State Journal of Medicine—for use of the diagram in my article "Preventive Aspects of Physical Fitness," in Vol. 64, No. 10, May 15, 1964.

Sports Illustrated—for the quotation from the article "The Soft American" by John F. Kennedy, December 26, 1960.

Dr. Jean Mayer—for the table from his *Nutrition in Clinical Medicine,* copyright © 1960.

Dr. Jean Mayer and Harper & Row—for the conclusion from the chapter "Exercise and Weight Control" in *Science and Medicine of Exercise and Sports.*

**ALL NAMES OF PATIENTS MENTIONED IN THIS BOOK
ARE FICTITIOUS.**

Contents

CHAPTER 1

Test Yourself

PROGRESS BRINGS BENEFITS. It also brings perils. Man has been on earth for more than 100,000 years, and yet in the last hundred years, a brief flash in the infinity of time, he has changed his environment in revolutionary fashion. He has moved from a life of hard physical activity to a life of inertia in which machines do the work. He has moved from the quiet of the countryside to the city with its ceaseless irritations.

Nowhere is this more true than in the United States. On the face of it we have benefited greatly by progress. We are the most prosperous nation in the world. We have a superabundance of automobiles, appliances, and other labor-saving devices. In medicine we have conquered tuberculosis, polio, diphtheria, and a host of other diseases. Yet at the same time progress also has brought perils of its own. We have so altered the physical balance of our lives that we are now beset by a new wave of degenerative diseases. We have become so physically inactive that underexercise, often in conjunction with over-irritation, has become the most serious threat to the health of Americans. Approximately one out of every two Americans is under-exercised, and you may be among them. If you are, you should be seriously concerned about your health. Under-exercise is a major factor in causing back pain and tension syndrome (stiff neck and headache), and even emotional instability, duodenal ulcers, diabetes, and heart disease.

These degenerative afflictions are known as the hypo-kinetic diseases, the sicknesses caused by insufficient exercise. These are the diseases of an advanced civilization, and only in the last ten or fifteen years have we started to cope with them. Fortunately there is a way for you, or the members of your family, to find out if you are underexercised and a potential target for disease. You can test yourself by taking the six simple tests shown below. These are known as the Kraus-Weber tests, and they are for everyone, regardless of age, height, or weight. Designed to test the key muscle groups in your body, they reveal whether or not you have the necessary strength to handle your own body weight and the flexibility to match your height.

Before you test yourself, make yourself comfortable. Take off your shoes. Try to put yourself in a relaxed frame of mind. Do not rush. Do not push. Do not strain. Simply take the tests as directed. If you have back trouble or any other health problems, check with your physician before taking these tests.

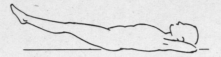

1. Lie flat on your back on the floor with your hands clasped behind your neck and with your legs straight and touching. Now keep your knees straight and lift your feet so that your heels are ten inches above the floor, as shown in the drawing. You pass this test if you can hold that position for ten seconds. This test shows if your hip flexors have sufficient strength.

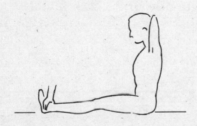

2. Lie flat on the floor again with your hands clasped behind your neck. Have someone hold down your legs by grasping the ankles as illustrated. If you live alone, hook your ankles under a heavy chair that won't topple. All right, now pass this test by rolling up into a sitting position. You pass if you can do one sit-up. This test reveals whether or not your hip flexors *and* stomach muscles combined are strong enough to handle your body weight.

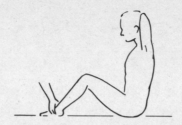

3. Once again, lie flat on the floor with your hands behind your neck, only this time have your knees flexed, heels close to buttocks. Make sure your ankles are held down. Now roll up into a sitting position again. This tests the strength of your stomach muscles.

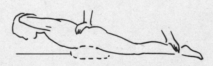

4. Turn over on your stomach. Put a pillow under your abdomen, clasp your hands behind your neck, and lie flat on the floor. Have your helper hold the lower half of your body steady by placing one hand in the small of the back and the other on your ankles. Now lift your trunk and hold it steady for ten seconds. This test reveals whether or not your back muscles are strong.

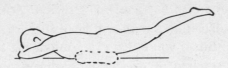

5. Stay on your stomach, fold your arms under your head, and make sure that the pillow is still under your abdomen. Have your helper hold your back steady with both hands. Now lift your legs up, be sure to keep your knees straight, and hold the position for ten seconds. This tests the strength of your low-back muscles.

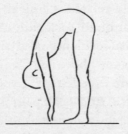

6. This is the last test. Stand up straight and make sure your feet are together. Now relax, lean over, and touch the floor with your finger tips without bending your knees. If you can pass this test, you have sufficient flexibility in your back muscles and hamstrings, the muscles in the back of your thighs. If you fail, it is because these muscles have become shortened and tense, not because your arms are too short or your legs too long.

11

These K-W tests are among the most important you can take to check your health. If you passed all six, you are meeting *the minimum levels of muscular fitness.* That is, you have sufficient strength and flexibility for your weight and height. But if you failed even one of the six tests, you are underexercised or overtensed and you need help. In fact, if you had difficulty passing any one of these tests, you should consider yourself below par. This may seem severe or unfair, but you would not be considered healthy if you had perfect vision and hearing, a good pulse rate, but an abnormal red-cell blood count.

This book is directed not only to anyone who is underexercised but also toward anyone already suffering from back pain, stiff neck, or tension. Back pain and underexercise are intimately related. Clinical studies show that more than 80 per cent of all back-pain cases are caused by underexercise. Clinical evidence also shows that if you failed one or more of the above tests, and do not yet have back pain, the odds are excellent that you will suffer from back pain in the future. And back pain is often merely the first of the hypokinetic diseases to strike the underexercised.

Back pain, or tension syndrome, is no joy. The pain can strike almost anywhere from the neck to the waist. It can be the pulsing throb of a tension headache so excruciating it is torture to try to focus your eyes; tense neck muscles can cause this. Tense neck and shoulder muscles can also cause a horrible stiff neck that makes it agony to turn from side to side. Some people, often those with desk jobs, suffer stabbing pain between the shoulder blades. But the worst of all is low back pain. A bad case of low back pain makes you think that you're crippled for life. If your muscles are weak and tense, low back pain can strike at any time. Suddenly all the tension that has been building up in your system seems to focus across the lower back, just above the buttocks. In an instant, as you go to turn or twist or to stoop or straighten up, muscles go into a wracking spasm. You cannot move. You are locked into position. You wonder what hit you. You wonder if you dare straighten up. You try to, and you immediately feel as though someone had stuck a knife in your spine. You try to get to a chair, and the pain increases even more. Finally you manage to lie down. When the pain is really piercing, you cannot get up. You can't move your legs. Even a slight shift in bed triggers the pain. For a day or two the pain persists. Then slowly it ebbs. At last you manage to hobble out of bed. Then the pain seems to go away, and you gingerly test your back. A week, a month, maybe two months later, the pain attacks again. This time it's worse. You wonder what's wrong. Nothing seems to help.

All this is very familiar to physicians; they hear it from patients all the time. But these patients can be helped, and you can be helped. If these patients had been in reasonable condition, if they could have passed the six K-W tests, probably they never would have needed help. If they had led more balanced lives, if they had exercised and exercised correctly, they would have felt fine. They would have had healthy backs, sound backs, fit backs, not sick backs, not muscularly deficient backs.

Let me give you a case in point of a sick-back sufferer who was warned five years ahead of time that he was bound to have trouble. I'll call him Pete Hamilton. He is a magazine staff writer, and we first met over the telephone when he called me at my country place. This was in 1955, and the K-W tests were "news" because of a report I had given to the then President, Dwight Eisenhower.

"I want to know all about the Kraus-Weber tests, what they mean, everything," said Mr. Hamilton over the phone. "If you don't mind, I'd like to fly up to see you today. I have to do the story quickly."

"All right," I said. "Come on up and we'll talk."

Pete Hamilton arrived that afternoon. He was a pleasant young man in his late twenties. He was of medium height and was just starting to run to fat. He was perhaps five or ten pounds overweight. But what really struck me about him was his intensity. He was all wound up. He exuded tension. In fact, when I met him at the airport, he was suffering from a tension headache. He said he didn't like to fly and that he had gotten the headache on the way up.

Well, everything went fine that day. I gave Mr. Hamilton all sorts of facts, and we talked and talked until ten or eleven that night. The next morning after we had breakfast he asked, "Would you mind putting me through the Kraus-Weber tests?"

"Not at all," I said. "I'd be delighted."

He took off his shoes and got down on the floor. I gave him the six tests. He had good strength; he had no trouble whatsoever moving his body weight. But as I had figured from watching him, he was tense. In fact, he was so tense that he failed the floor-touch test, which gauges the flexibility of the back muscles and the hamstrings. When I say

14

he failed, I mean he really failed. Strain and grunt as he did, he couldn't get his finger tips to within six inches of the floor. I checked his hamstrings, and they felt as unyielding as piano wire.

I said, "If I ever saw a candidate for back pain, you're it. You're simply too tense. Tell me, what do you do for exercise?"

"Nothing," he said.

"Don't you exercise at all?" I asked. "Don't you ever work out in a gym? Don't you swim?"

"No, Doctor," he said. "I was as active as could be when I was a kid. But when I reached sixteen or seventeen, I started to study a lot and I just sort of let exercise slide by. Besides, I'm very busy with my work, and in addition to that I live in the city, and unless I happen to live across the street from a tennis court or a pool, I just can't be bothered to take the time. I feel okay. I know I'm tense, but that's me. I'm just naturally a tense person."

"That may be you," I said, "but that shouldn't be you. Tension is very bad for your muscles. It shortens them. That's why you can't even get close to the floor with your finger tips. I strongly recommend that you start a regular exercise program to relieve the tension and make you relaxed."

"I'm sorry, Doctor," Pete said, "but I'm just too rushed to do that."

"You're wrong," I said. "But you run your life your own way and see what happens."

Pete Hamilton went off and wrote his story. I read it, and he had done an accurate job. He told everyone what

15

was wrong with underexercised and overstimulated living, and he told everyone why they should exercise. Of course, he didn't write in the story that he himself was "too busy" to exercise. Pete was one of those people who believe in fitness for everyone but himself.

I didn't see Pete Hamilton until five years later, and when I did he limped into the clinic, bent over at the waist, a look of agony on his face. He smiled ruefully and slowly backed into a chair to tell me what had happened.

"After I saw you, Doctor," Pete began, "I moved out to the Midwest to work as a correspondent. Then my wife and I moved to the West Coast. Two years ago we moved back to New York. We bought a house up in the country, and I began commuting. About a month after we moved in, I happened to use the car to go to the office. It was raining when I started back home, and to make the story brief, I went into a skid, a bad skid, on the parkway. There were cars coming at me from the opposite direction, and since I didn't want to slam into them head on, I yanked the wheel in the opposite direction, and I really went for a ride. The car turned around three times before stopping, but the odd thing was that I was okay. So I thought. I didn't have a scratch, although the car was smashed up against a guardrail. But the next day at home—I had the day off—I felt a slight pain in the lower back. It bothered me, but I didn't think it was bad. Then, a few minutes later, I went to pick up a piece of paper from the kitchen floor, and, wham, I fell down. It was as though someone had swung an ax into the base of my spine. I was flat on my face and I couldn't

16

move my legs. I stayed there for a half hour until my wife found me. She called the volunteer fire department. They came, put me in a stretcher—boy, did that hurt—and took me upstairs to bed. My wife called our doctor, and he called an ambulance. I spent a week in the hospital in traction.

"I wore a brace when I came home, but the back just got worse. Two months later it went out again. This time I spent three weeks in bed. I just couldn't face the hospital again. At Christmas my back went out again. In the spring I was laid up for a month. Two months ago the back went out again. Now I am desperate. My doctor says I may need a spinal fusion, but before he operates, he wants you to see me. Doctor, is there *anything* you can do?"

When I finished examining him, I said, "Let's forget about surgery now. When you skidded in that car, your back muscles couldn't relax. They had no give to meet this emergency. They had been shortened by constant tension, and you tore a muscle slightly. Since you are tense, the muscles have never had a chance to relax and heal the tear. This may be all that's ailing you. Now here's what we will try. First, get rid of the brace. It will only weaken your stomach muscles, and the examination shows you have all the strength you need. What you need are relaxing exercises, exercises to stretch your hamstrings and back muscles. These will help those shortened muscles to become flexible and resilient. You will get rid of the tension. Do not do any bending or lifting for the present. Come to the clinic three times a week for the next two months. The

17

therapist will give you certain exercises to do. Learn how to do them properly, then we'll examine you again. Above all, don't worry."

Three months later Pete Hamilton was fine. He could walk erect. He could touch the floor with his finger tips. The pain was gone. The tension was gone. Soon he was on his own, doing a daily set of prescribed exercises that he had learned in our clinic. Not long ago Pete Hamilton called to ask me to treat a friend. During the conversation he said, "Doctor, I want you to know that I feel just great. I do the exercises every day, and I have no pain. I run, I swim, I chop two or three cords of wood a winter, but above all, I don't feel tense all the time. If I start to feel tense, I'll take a half hour, shut out the world, and do my exercises. After that I'm as relaxed as can be."

I'm glad that Pete is fine now. I'm only sorry that he did not avoid all the pain and anguish that he had been warned about. But you don't have to do anything as dramatic as wrecking your car to hurt your back. That sudden jab of pain which can lock your muscles tight, can strike at any time. You may stoop over to pick a flower and suddenly your back muscles are in spasm. Back pain may strike when you start to get up from a chair or when you're tying your shoelaces or swinging a golf club or a tennis racket or simply turning a doorknob. When it strikes, you know it. And when it strikes once, it will come back, again and again, unless you do something about it.

Severe back pain is one of the most common medical complaints today, and yet it is one of the least understood. Why? Because the underlying causes of back pain are so subtle and so insidious. Being out of shape has become one of the accepted facts of American life, and most people are in such poor shape that the abnormal is thought of as the normal.

Back pain occurs most often for two reasons. First of all, millions of Americans are underexercised. We live in a sedentary age. Progress has robbed us of our physical heritage. Fifty or a hundred years ago you would have had to do hard physical tasks in the ordinary routine of living. You would have walked, run, ridden a horse, chopped wood, plowed fields, or done household chores that were muscularly demanding. But look at the easy life you lead now. Instead of walking or running, you drive a car. And the car has power steering—you don't even have to move your arms. Instead of climbing stairs, you take an elevator. When you want heat, you don't shovel coal; you simply turn up a thermostat. When you do laundry, you just dump it in a machine. And when you want to dry it, you dump it in another. You do not have to wash dishes; a machine does it for you. There are appliances all over the house. Mixers have done away with the egg beater. Vacuum cleaners have supplanted the broom. There are electric razors and even electric toothbrushes. When you ski, you take a chair lift up the hill; when you play golf, you ride a cart. In short, you lead a mechanized push-button life, and so do many other Americans. And millions are underexercised as a result.

The other contributing factor is tension. In years past you would have worked off your tension doing physical tasks. Nowadays, not only do you not do physical work, but you live in a hectic age of crowded cities and suburbs as well. You are overstimulated and over-irritated every day. There is the rush to the office in the morning, the annoyance of traffic jams, late trains and slow buses, the constant chatter of TV commercials, the pesky appliance that won't work, the continuous ring of the telephone, the loud radio next door. When you are irritated by any one of these or similar annoyances, muscles actually tense in preparation for action. Repeated irritations will make the muscles stiff and short. The next time the phone rings or a commercial blares, notice how you stiffen and tense. Think of how many times a day countless irritations like this occur.

On top of these external irritants there are internal irritations. You may be worried and under strain because of a personal problem, which can be anything from money worries to unhappy sex relations. These internal problems can make you tense just from thinking about them. Your emotions affect your muscles. The two are bound together, not only physiologically but semantically. The word "emotion" literally means to move. Your muscles reflect your emotional problems. When you say that a certain problem is "a pain in the neck" or "a headache," or that so-and-so is "a pain in the behind," you are speaking the truth.

The underexercised and over-irritated life we lead today is especially bad for children, who should be developing strong and resilient muscles for adulthood. Children rarely suffer from back pain, but youngsters with weak and tense muscles will be lucky if they suffer only back pain when they reach their twenties. When you grew up a generation ago, you led a far more vigorous childhood than the majority of youngsters do today. If your muscles act up, you at least have a base on which to build: the muscles you developed as a youngster. But the situation has gotten worse in the last twenty years. For one thing, you didn't grow up with television, on which children today spend hours. Television has a doubly bad effect on youngsters. A child gets no physical benefit whatsoever from watching television. Also, a child gets tense from television. His muscles will become tense and shortened, and he will assume poor posture. Instead of getting tense watching cowboys and Indians indoors, a youngster should be outdoors getting rid of tension playing cowboys and Indians.

Back pain may begin early in life, in the twenties or thirties. It hits men and women alike. It can hit men and women at any time, but there are two periods in a woman's life when she is most likely to suffer. These are after she has a child and when she is in menopause. A woman in change of life is prone to back pain because she is under tension and because her hormonal balance is upset. A woman who has just had a child is in danger because of all the lifting she has to do. She also may be under stress. Take the case of Jane C., a very attractive suburban mother. As a young girl, Jane grew up in the city. She enjoyed good health, but she never was physically active.

Jane got married when she was twenty-two. She and her husband moved to a suburban town, and they were very happy. A year after they were married Jane gave birth to a boy. A month before the baby was born, she woke up one night in bed with a dull ache in the middle of the lower part of her back. Her husband rubbed the ache for her, and she went back to sleep. But when Jane woke up in the morning, the ache was still there, and she dragged herself through the day. She didn't feel irritable; she just felt blah. She thought the ache came from being in the late stages of pregnancy, and she was right. The only trouble was that she also thought it would go away after she had the baby, and she didn't say anything to her obstetrician.

But when Jane came home from the hospital with the baby, the dull ache had become sharp pain. And it wasn't just in the lower back either; it smarted sharply down into her left buttock. She tried to put the pain out of her mind as she looked after the infant, nursing him, changing him, feeding him, but as the months went by the pain grew in severity.

One night, when the baby was about four months old, Jane couldn't sleep. Now the pain was shooting down her left leg. From the lower back to above the back of her knee, it was one pulsing throb. She found it impossible to get back to sleep, and the next morning she made an appointment with her obstetrician. He examined her and found nothing wrong.

The pain continued, and Jane called her general practitioner. It was the same story. When the baby was a year and a half old and Jane was at her wit's end, the pain suddenly stopped.

Two years later Jane became pregnant again. Two months before this baby was due the back pain returned. This time the pain began by shooting down her left leg. She had a restless, irritable pregnancy. She was glad to see that the baby, another son, was fine and healthy, but right after she returned home with him she started to resent him. She hated herself for feeling this way, but the more she had to tend the baby, the more she resented him because the pain was just too much and she blamed the baby for her discomfort. Now she couldn't even get to sleep at night. She tossed fitfully for hours, and when she did lapse into sleep, it was the sleep of the exhausted. Once again she saw her obstetrician. Again he could find nothing wrong. Her G.P. finally referred her to our clinic.

We examined her carefully, had X-rays taken, and finally put her through the K-W tests described at the beginning of this chapter. After Jane took them, I looked over her medical history once more and then told her, "You have nothing to worry about as long as you follow directions. Let me tell you what the trouble is. First of all, as you know even better than I do, your lower back muscles are very, very tender. That is because they are tight. Why are they tight? Not because you're a tense person—although you are starting to get tense from worrying about your back—but because you don't have any strength in your stomach muscles. The pain started in the eighth month of your first pregnancy, and you got it because your weak stomach muscles forced you to carry the weight of the child with your back muscles. Your stomach muscles were weak because you never had made them strong when you were a child. Now, the pain got worse after you had the baby because you had to bend over and lift him, you had to carry him, and you had to change his diapers. Then, when he was a year and a half old, he could walk by himself, and so you didn't have to lift him as much and the pain subsided.

"But with the second pregnancy and the second child, the pain came back. You have simply put too much of a load on your back muscles. Now, what you have to do is to build up the strength of those stomach muscles, and you are going to do that by following a daily exercise program. At first you will need more rest and a corset for your back—until your muscles get strong enough to support it unaided."

That day Jane began exercising to strengthen her stomach muscles. She did the exercises every day, and her back pain gradually subsided. By doing exercises prescribed to correct the weakness that had made her back unbearable, Jane was able to avoid future difficulty.

Often tension has a great deal to do with back pain. In fact, tension, or lack of flexibility, is responsible for more attacks of back pain than any other single cause. Even if you are physically strong, you can be struck with a bad back, caused by tension, that will render you helpless. If you are over-irritated, overstimulated or even overeager, your tense mental state will be reflected in your muscles, and unless you exercise properly, the tension will accumulate. This can happen to a strong person over a period of years. Here is the case of an ex-college football star whom I'll call Steve B.

Steve grew up in a poor family. He had to hustle for everything he earned. He was a big, strapping boy, and he was tough. When he was seventeen, he was six foot two, weighed 220 pounds, and was an A student. Above all, he could really play football, and scouts from all over the country were after him. He not only had the muscle they were looking for, but he also had an intense desire to win. His childhood had made him extremely competitive.

Steve got many offers to play football. Some schools offered cash on the line, but Steve was looking for the school that would give him the best education. He finally accepted a scholarship at a prestigious eastern school. For three years he played varsity ball. He did extremely well, but he did even better in his studies. Upon graduation he joined a large industrial firm as a trainee. In five years he was a plant manager. But in the course of time Steve changed without realizing it. He was so busy that he gave up running every morning and working out in the gym. When he was only in his mid-thirties, he was made a vice-president. He was busier than ever. There were business lunches and social meetings. His work became his life. He grew tense without knowing it. His weight began to creep up on him. He was 240, then 250. He carried it well, but he was running to flab. He didn't exercise at all, but everyone who knew of him thought he was as strong and tough as he had been in the days when he was the terror of the football field. No one thought this more than Steve himself. He still had that strong competitive drive, but now it was devoted to business instead of football. The bathroom scale told Steve he was getting heavier, and his panting breath told him he was getting out of shape, but Steve paid no heed. The changes were slow and subtle; Steve accepted tension as a fate common to all executives who led the busy life he did. Like a lot of people, he accepted the abnormal as normal. Sure he was tense, but wasn't everybody else?

Then Steve's back "went out." It was not at all dramatic. It was simply the response to the inevitable. It was a gray January day, and snow had fallen all night long. Steve had an important appointment, and he had to drive to the office. The snow was two feet deep, and he had to shovel a pathway from his garage to the street. As he shoveled hurriedly, it seemed like hard work compared with what it had been in the past, but, always the competitor, Steve battled to get the job done. When he had finished shoveling, he felt a muscle twinge low in his back. He paid no attention to it. However, when he arrived at the office, he found it difficult to get out of the car. As he tried to straighten up behind the wheel, he felt a sudden stabbing pain in the lower back. He finally had to clamber out in a stooped position.

Steve struggled through the day and managed to drive home. The pain was worse when he went to bed. He stayed in bed for a couple of days and then came to our clinic for help.

Examination showed that his stomach muscles and hip flexors were weak and that his hamstrings were stiff and tense. When I told him this, he protested, "Doctor, I'm an athlete. I played football. I'm as strong as an ox."

"You *were* an athlete," I replied, "and if you're as strong as an ox, why can't you shovel a driveway without straining your back? You've changed. Your body has changed. You were strong, but that was fifteen years ago. You've been up to your neck in business. You don't exercise. You're extremely tense. Do you think that because you once played football when you were young that you're fine now? You must face facts."

He didn't say a word.

"Now look," I said, "there is no reason for you to become despondent. You're not permanently crippled. You just have to take stock of your condition. I can tell you what you should do, and it is up to you to cooperate if you want to get better."

First Steve needed treatment to relieve his pain. Two weeks later he embarked on therapeutic exercises designed to strengthen his stomach muscles and hip flexors and loosen his tight hamstrings. Within three months he returned to his former strength and flexibility, and he lost fourteen pounds besides. The tension ebbed. He felt fine. To this day he has continued exercises. Steve has given himself a new lease on life.

And now what about you? What can you do? You can do quite a lot. First of all, you can exercise. You can and should exercise *correctly,* and doing this will help correct any deficiency you may have. But first a word of caution.

In recent years there has been a growing interest in exercise. There are exercise and fitness books by the dozen. Some of them even offer good exercises. But the question is, are these exercises for you? They may not be. Before

you ever start exercising on a regular basis, you have to
know what your individual needs are. The majority of
people do not know what their needs are, yet they buy
exercise books and go at the exercises with a vengeance.
In doing this they often injure themselves. As a matter of
fact, we regularly see two or three new patients a week who
have injured themselves because they were faithfully doing
the exercises handed down for everyone in one very popular exercise book. Not all of us are alike in our muscular
problems, and all of us cannot do the same set of exercises
without risk of injury. You may lack strong stomach
muscles. Your friend, Joe, has strong stomach muscles but
no flexibility in his low back muscles and hamstrings. Your
friend, Betty, lacks flexibility in her hamstrings and has
weak hip flexors as well. All of you cannot go and do the
same set of exercises from the same book and benefit because you may all have different problems. At least one of
you is likely to get hurt. For instance, if you are tense and
you start doing isometric exercises, the latest exercise fad,
you are going to have even more tension, and you can hurt
yourself badly. Isometric exercising calls upon you to tense
a muscle without actually producing any movement of the
limbs or body. Enthusiasts claim that if you do this tensing
just a few minutes a day, you will get in excellent shape.
This is not borne out by fact. Physical medicine has been
aware of isometric exercises for a long time, and while the
exercises will increase strength to a certain point, the gain
in strength will then level off, and much more exercising
of an entirely different kind is then needed to produce a

28

really strong muscle. But the potential danger in isometrics is that they are likely to make your muscles stiff and tense —the last thing you want them to be.

Whether or not an exercise book recommends isometrics or some other form of exercise, you should be wary, even if you already are in excellent condition. Most of these books cannot consider your own particular needs. Instead they blithely give exercises for everyone. I would no more think of telling everyone to do the same set of exercises than your family doctor would tell all his patients, no matter whether they had a broken leg, sinus trouble, or heart disease, to take the same medicine. Let me cite a very recent case as an example.

Robert F. came to see us with severe pain in his upper back, between the shoulder blades. Mr. F. likes to be physically active, so when he became very busy at the office and had no time for the tennis he ordinarily played to stay in shape, he started doing exercises to make up for the lack. He bought a very popular book, a best-seller, in fact, read it, and started doing the exercises every day. One exercise called for him to lie on the floor and arch his upper back quickly. He started with ten repetitions of this and worked his way up to twenty a day when the pain started. But he mistakenly thought there was something wrong with himself, so he worked his way up to forty a day, until the pain just refused to allow him to continue. When Mr. F. came to the clinic, his upper back muscles were in severe spasm. I told him to cease his exercises immediately. It took several days to relieve the pain, and then we gave him an exercise program that would relax and stretch the upper back muscles instead of making them tense and stiff. He did, and the tension subsided.

In brief, exercises must be prescribed individually to treat a specific condition. First, you must know what is wrong. You can find out what is wrong with your key posture muscles by taking the Kraus-Weber tests. Each one of those six tests is for a key muscle group in your body. For instance, if you are unable to touch the floor with your finger tips (Test 6), your lower back muscles and hamstrings are stiff and tense. Therefore you should do relaxation, limbering, and stretching exercises. If you are unable to roll up to a sitting position with your knees flexed (Test 3), your stomach muscles need strengthening exercises. It may be that you will need to do both strengthening and flexibility exercises at the same time. What you need to do, and what you can do through exercise, is spelled out completely in Chapter 6.

But exercise alone is not the answer. Proper exercise is an important key to good health, but it is only one of several keys. If you take the proper approach, you can stop the effect of tension before it even starts. You can do the same for your children either at home or in school. You can learn what sports are best for you and for them. Some sports and activities are sure to be tension builders. Others are not only tension relievers but help improve your heart and blood vessels. You should know the difference. You may be overweight and on a diet. Is your diet really necessary? It may not be.

In short, you must study yourself, your mind, your daily

routine, your work and living habits, and your emotional attitudes as well as your body. By all means find out where you are physically weak or strong, but also try to learn what actually prompts tension or pain. You must try to find out about yourself. Once you do, you can approach your problems with a sense of purposeful direction.

ADVANTAGES OF THE PHYSICALLY
ACTIVE AS COMPARED TO SEDENTARY

ACTIVE		SEDENTARY
LOW	WEIGHT	HIGH
LOW	BLOOD PRESSURE	HIGH
LOW	PULSE RATE	HIGH
LOW	NEURO-MUSCULAR TENSION	HIGH
HIGH	MUSCLE STRENGTH AND FLEXIBILITY	LOW
HIGH	BREATHING CAPACITY	LOW
HIGH	ADRENO-CORTICAL RESERVE	LOW
HIGH	TIREDNESS LEVEL	LOW
HIGH	EMOTIONAL STABILITY	LOW
HIGH	HEART STRENGTH	LOW
LATE	AGING	EARLY

CHAPTER 2

Why Back Pain Comes

THE TREATMENT of back pain has always offered a fertile field for the quack. America's first notorious quack, Elisha Perkins, who died in 1799, believed—and he was apparently sincere about this—that certain metals could yank pain from the body. He invented a device called a "tractor," consisting of two short metal rods, which he sold for $25. A patient was supposed to work the tractor by running it down over the pain.

Generally you can spot a quack because he usually has something to sell. It might be a magic board that rests against your back, or it might be a "healing" belt. Whatever it is, it is always a gimmick, it costs money, it is guaranteed to cure, and it is worthless.

There are several reasons why quacks have had a field day with back-pain sufferers. First of all, back pain is a relatively new problem. In the past back pain was rare, and when it did occur, it was usually caused by serious disease or injury, such as ruptured discs. Help was sought through the normal approaches of medicine and surgery. It is only recently that "everybody" has started having a bad back, but unless a patient is afflicted with a mechanically unstable spine or a serious disease, the ailment is considered unimportant. In recent decades medical attention has focused on major surgery and research, and if back pain cannot be related to a major disability, it is considered to be of little significance. It is no wonder then that many physicians are uninterested in what might be called the garden variety of backache.

In the past few years, however, increasing numbers of physicians and surgeons have begun to realize that garden-variety back pain is of a complex origin and must be regarded as one of the major ailments of a mechanized society. But instead of turning to braces and surgery, which are necessary only in relatively few cases, these physicians and surgeons have returned to one of the oldest and most valuable tools of medicine: therapeutic exercise. Compared with surgery, therapeutic exercise may seem undramatic, but in case after case its use has been extremely rewarding.

A century ago exercise was prescribed quite widely by physicians. In Sweden, Pehr Henrik Ling, a student of anatomy, developed a system of therapeutic exercises that was used by physicians in most countries. One of his pupils, Dr. George H. Taylor, brought his ideas to the United States and wrote a widely consulted book, *Exposition of the Swedish Movement Cure*. Exercise was regarded both as a way of promoting health and as a way of correcting bodily defects. But then, with the dramatic strides in medicine, particularly in surgery and in the development of drugs, which came toward the end of the nineteenth century,

34

exercise began to lose out not only in medicine but in the schools as well. By the 1920s the medical aspect of exercise had been all but forgotten in the United States. Of course, at the time we were still a somewhat physically vigorous people—progress had not yet robbed us of daily physical activity.

I came upon the value of exercise through happenstance more than thirty years ago, when I was a young hospital intern in surgery. One of my jobs at the time was to serve on emergency duty, taking care of fractures. In addition to this I had to review the results of hundreds and hundreds of cases involving wrist fractures. I had to find out how the patients were doing. Had their breaks healed? Did they still feel pain? What did follow-up X-rays show? As I went through case after case, a common pattern began to emerge: the patients who made the best recoveries were those who had exercised the most after the fracture. It made no difference if their fractures had originally been worse than those suffered by others. The fact was that the recovery rate of patients who exercised was better and quicker than that of patients who did little or no exercise.

After I reported this to our chief surgeon, the hospital started reviewing the results of other fracture cases. The findings were similar: exercise was decidedly helpful. As a result, the hospital decided to start a special department where all fracture patients could receive exercises. Shortly afterward any patient who had spent any time at all in bed in the hospital was given special exercises to re-establish muscular strength and flexibility through systematic training.

In those early years—and this is long before the six K-W tests were even thought of—I learned a great deal from an athlete, coach, and exercise teacher named Heinz Kowalski, who ran a local gym. Originally he had been a circus acrobat, and he was an artist in conditioning the people, mostly athletes, who came to his gym for help. As I watched Kowalski, I began to see that some of his techniques could be used to treat the sick or the physically deficient. A specific instance comes to mind. Kowalski and I used to work out together at the gym, and one day I asked him, "How is it that you never send anyone with a sprain to the hospital? You send us fracture patients, but I don't know of one person you've sent us with a sprain."

"Oh," Kowalski said in his calm way, "you wouldn't know how to treat a sprain."

"What do you mean?" I asked. "We're physicians, surgeons. We certainly know how to treat sprains."

"I don't know about that," he said. "When you get your hands on someone with a sprained shoulder or a sprained ankle, you wrap him up in bandages and keep him immobilized for weeks. I don't do that. In my family we had to perform every night in the circus. We couldn't be out of action. When we got sprains, we performed in spite of them. We knew what to do. The minute we got a sprain, we treated it with hot steam, alcohol applications, and movement. The pain went away and we could go on with our performance. The exercise did it good. The next day we were fine."

I was interested in what he had to say. Obviously hot steam and alcohol have their drawbacks—it is easy, as I

36

found out the hard way, to scald yourself—and so I looked about for something else that would ease the pain and allow movement. After trial and error I found it—ethyl chloride spray. It is often more effective than ice or heat. When this fluid, which should be used only by physicians, is sprayed on the skin, it evaporates quickly and dulls the sense of pain by freezing. The pain must be lessened so the injured part can be moved. The movement is essential to the healing process; otherwise the effect of the ethyl chloride is temporary. Nowadays many physicians find ethyl chloride most helpful in treating sprains and strains and in relieving the pain of back muscles in spasm.

Later on Harold Anson Bruce, the great track coach, also taught me certain principles. Bruce was a living lesson in conditioning. He showed that you don't have to run to flab at the age of forty. When he was seventy, he competed in the national cross-country tryouts and placed fifteenth in a large field.

In 1940 I had the good fortune to work with Dr. Sonja Weber in the Posture Clinic of Columbia-Presbyterian Hospital in New York City. This clinic had been established to treat children who had posture problems. Some of the youngsters were afflicted with injuries or birth deformities, but most of our young patients were well and their bones and functions were considered normal; they had been sent to us simply because they had "poor posture."

We spent many hours in detailed examinations of the youngsters. We photographed them, made line drawings, and conducted all sorts of studies, trying to find out more about the muscles of these otherwise normal children who had bad posture. At first we had little success. We noticed that the children quickly learned to assume good posture when examined or observed but then slipped back into poor posture when they thought no one was looking.

After more investigation it occurred to us that poor posture was often the result of a muscular inability to move properly. To check on proper movement, we decided to measure the strength and flexibility of the back, stomach, and hip muscles used to hold the body erect. We spent several years experimenting with muscle measurements and muscle tests. We prescribed various corrective exercises. From time to time we would compare the results of these exercises with physical changes in the patients.

Finally we agreed on a battery of fifteen muscle tests, of which the six key tests later became known as the Kraus-Weber tests. Using them, we could quickly and easily determine which muscles were weak or tense. We could understand why children slouched, why their stomachs stuck out, why they had round shoulders or sway-backs. After giving the children the tests and noting which ones they failed, we would then give each child a specific set of exercises to correct his or her particular condition. Those who exercised according to our prescriptions often improved. Those who did the exercises and then stopped reverted to previous defects as their muscles deteriorated.

In 1944 Dr. Barbara Stimson asked Dr. Weber and me to participate in a special back clinic she had organized at Columbia-Presbyterian Hospital, under the auspices of Drs. William Darrach and Clay Ray Murray. Later on the work was pursued at Dr. Howard Rusk's Institute for Physical Medicine and Rehabilitation at New York University. Dr. Stimson had started the clinic to find the cause for the ever-increasing number of back-pain sufferers. Back pain had become a problem in the armed services, in industry, and in everyday life. The clinic staff at Columbia-Presbyterian Hospital included orthopedic surgeons, internists, neurosurgeons, psychiatrists, and neurologists. X-ray and routine laboratory tests were made of every back-pain patient. In more than 80 per cent of the cases, nothing at all abnormal was found. Dr. Weber and I were then asked to study the muscular efficiency of these patients. We decided to use the six key tests we had developed for children at the Posture Clinic. Upon administering the tests to the back patients, we at once discovered that not only were they weak and tense but we could see exactly where the deficiencies were. Exercises were prescribed to fit each individual case.

The benefits of the exercises were soon evident. The patients who did them faithfully often found relief from back pain in a few weeks or months. Those who did not exercise continued to suffer. Their suffering was understandable, because muscles are healthy only when they are properly used.

It took us only a little more time to realize something else, that we had not only discovered an effective way of treating and relieving muscular back pain, but, more importantly perhaps, we had found, in the six Kraus-Weber tests, *a way of predicting potential back trouble*. We discovered this when we began giving the Kraus-Weber tests

39

LOW BACK PAIN
Over 80% of low back pain is due to muscular deficiency

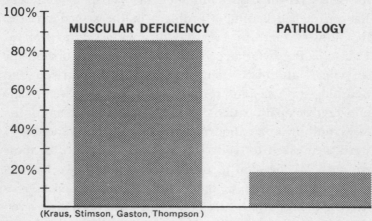

(Kraus, Stimson, Gaston, Thompson)

80% of low back pain is due to lack of adequate physical activity. (H. Kraus, B. Stimson, S. Gaston, W. Thompson).

to "healthy" people. Even though these people were considered well and had no pain, we often found that a person who failed even one of the six Kraus-Weber tests was a prime candidate for back trouble.

Dr. Weber and I both began to speculate about the general causes of back pain. We were very aware of the fact that people from all walks of life, from the armed forces to industry, were coming up with complaints. Discussing the problem back and forth, we wondered if many people had become weak and tense because now they were leading lives that were largely sedentary. In order to determine whether or not sedentary living habits were actually at the root of back trouble, we decided to test American school children and compare them with European school children who lacked such "benefits" of progress as television sets and automobiles. In 1952 we tested more than 5,000 healthy American children between the ages of six and sixteen in a half dozen urban and suburban areas in this country. These children, mind you, had all the care and medicine that an affluent society could give them.

These youngsters did poorly on the Kraus-Weber tests. They were amazingly weak and tense. Then we went to other less mechanized countries. In Austria, Italy, and Switzerland we tested about 3,000 children in the same age group. The difference was startling. Very few were weak or tense. In brief, we found:

> that 57.9 per cent of the American children failed one or more of the six tests, while only 8.7 per cent of the European children failed.

> that 44.3 per cent of the American children failed the flexibility test, while only 7.8 per cent of the European children failed.

> that 35.7 per cent of the American children failed one or more of the five strength tests, while only 1.1 per cent of the European children failed.

Realizing that we had important facts to reveal to both physicians and physical educators, we presented our findings at the annual meeting of the New York State Medical Society in 1954. The reception was somewhat cool, but it was warm compared with the chilly welcome we got at the annual meeting of the American Association for Health, Physical Education and Recreation. The physical educators politely applauded but simply refused to admit there was a problem.

We carried on our work. We continued our clinical studies of back patients and accumulated evidence that back pain was only one of the ailments afflicting the under-exercised. We began to see, as we pieced our data together bit by bit, that many back patients were sick in other ways. They were emotionally upset or under strain; they suffered from "tension," ulcers, and headaches. We then started to survey medical literature to discover if other "sedentary diseases" besides back pain had been found.

We discovered a wealth of material. We found that the protective value of exercise and physical activity extended to much more than muscles alone. Besides back pain, underexercise was correlated with coronary heart disease, duodenal ulcers, diabetes, obesity, "tension" and emotional instability.

Some of the findings were fascinating. Two British researchers, Doctors J. A. Heady and J. N. Morris, found that death from coronary heart disease occurs twice as often among the physically inactive as it does among the active. A striking example of this was a comparison study they made of drivers and conductors on double-decker buses in London. The drivers, who had to sit behind the wheel all day, were more than twice as susceptible to coronary heart disease than were their far more active colleagues, the conductors, who spent the working day climbing up and down the stairs of the buses. On the following page is a graph of Morris and Heady's findings.

Medical researchers had also found that the physically inactive person has high neuromuscular tension, high blood pressure, high pulse rate, less vital breathing capacity, and low adrenocortical reserve. Diabetes, too, is reported to have a high incidence among the physically inactive. Dr. Jean Mayer of Harvard has done significant work on the close relationship between overweight and underexercise, showing that exercise often has more effect on your weight than does your diet. (I have more to say about this in Chapter 9.) Dr. Lloyd Appleton of the U.S.

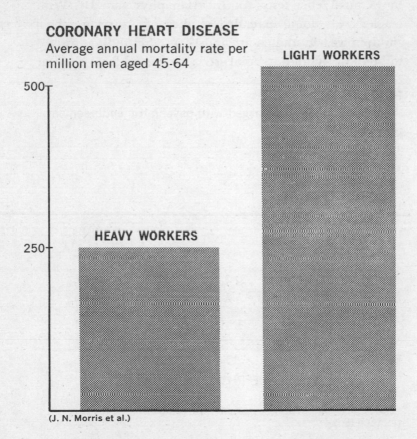

CORONARY HEART DISEASE
Average annual mortality rate per million men aged 45-64

LIGHT WORKERS

HEAVY WORKERS

500

250

(J. N. Morris et al.)

Military Academy at West Point discovered that 12.9 per cent of the cadets who finished in the lowest category on the Academy's physical-fitness test received psychiatric discharges. By contrast, no psychiatric difficulties were encountered in the most physically fit cadets.

At the same time that we were looking into the medical literature on the diseases caused by underexercise, we started getting reports from abroad on follow-up studies of the Kraus-Weber tests. An Austrian physician, Dr. Willi Nagler, was doing extended studies of Austrian school children we had studied previously, and his findings proved to be most significant. As Austria recovered from the war

PSYCHIATRIC
West Point cadets discharged with psychiatric endorsement

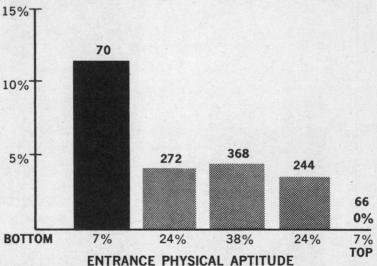

(Dr. Lloyd Appleton)

Lack of physical fitness goes parallel with emotional difficulties. (L. Appleton)

44

and moved into an era of prosperity, complete with television, automobiles, and appliances, the rate of failure on the K-W tests almost doubled.

Like the American youngsters, the Austrian children were starting to pay the penalties of progress by becoming underexercised. Reports came in from all over the world and, basically, they showed that physical fitness declined with mechanization and urbanization. Failure rates on tests shot up as a country became more prosperous. As the most prosperous nation in the world, the United States was in an ignominious position. It had—and still has—the most physically unfit youngsters. In tests administered by the Asian Foundation, Pakistani youngsters also rated much higher than their American counterparts. This was also true in Japan where researchers at Kyushu University studied 6,000 children.

These facts were disputed by physical educators. They declared the tests "invalid" and the findings inconclusive, even though they could not offer logical reasons for their opposition. In time the American Association for Health, Physical Education and Recreation composed their own test based on the movements of 5,000 American children. The test included running, jumping, and throwing a softball, and an average standard was established for the average child in different age groups. The test was then given in school systems all across the country, and most of them, of course, could happily state that their children were meeting the average standards.

No one seemed concerned that these "average" standards might not be up to standards in other countries until two physical educators, W. R. Campbell and R. H. Pohndorf, gave the test to 10,000 British boys and girls. Excluding the softball throw, the British youngsters scored 24 per cent higher than American youngsters.

Dr. Weber and I decided to study a group of adult Americans who were, almost by definition, physically inactive. We picked psychoanalysts, who sat in their offices all day listening to their patients. We followed case histories of twenty-six analysts with back pain from two to ten years, and we sent out hundreds of questionnaires to members of the American Psychoanalytical Association. Here is what we found:

We got clear answers to our questionnaires from 423 psychoanalysts. Of these, 144 exercised regularly and had no complaint of back pain; 107 did not exercise and did have pain; 47 analysts had back pain that was relieved by exercise; 52 had pain despite physical activity; 29 did not exercise and had no pain; 44 had disc trouble. The results were even clearer with the twenty-six analysts we personally studied. We prescribed exercises and encouraged them to move around for five minutes between patients. Our most recent follow-up survey reveals that of the twenty-six analysts, seven had no pain whatsoever, eighteen had definite relief, and one still had pain. This analyst, we later learned, had stopped his exercise therapy.

As we delved further and further into medical research on the underexercised, I could not help but recall that in the past physicians often told patients who were getting overweight that they should become more active, that they should chop wood, run, and even climb mountains. But in recent years too many physicians, it seemed, were giving overweight patients a diet—crash, gradual, or otherwise—

and said little, if anything, about exercise. I still remember a book that proclaims: "Exercise Is Bosh." Indeed, not long ago *The New York Times* Sunday Magazine Section carried an article by, of all people, a physician saying the same thing. None of these writings, and there are many others, are substantiated by facts.

In any event, the idea that underexercise was responsible, in whole or in part, for many ills was regarded as extremely radical in medical circles as recently as ten years ago. This I found when my associates and I presented our findings at the 1955 annual meeting of the American Medical Association.

We used the term hypokinetic disease to describe all the ailments—from back pain to heart trouble—induced at least in part by underexercise. Hypokinetic comes from the Greek, and by hypokinetic disease we mean all the sicknesses prompted by insufficient motion. Nowadays hypokinetic disease is becoming a most respectable medical term —you even see United States Government posters saying: "Fight Hypokinesia"—but at the time it was really Greek to most people.

True, we won a prize for the exhibit we presented on "hypokinetic disease," but most of the audience did not believe in exercise at all, and they were practically shouting at me when discussing my paper.

Among other things, my associates and I were accused of being unpatriotic. We were told, of all things, that we were maligning American athletes. Then one of the audience got up and said that we were wrong about American youngsters being weak and tense, because he happened to have a three-year-old boy he could not follow around the house. I suppose he considered this clinical evidence. His baby, he declared in ringing tones, was more active and faster than he was. I could only congratulate him on having such a healthy child; politeness forbade my commenting on the underexercised father.

There was one physician in the audience, however, who stood up and agreed with us wholeheartedly. This physician was Dr. Jessie Wright, who had been in charge of several children's clinics for many years, and she could bear out what we had found. She, too, felt that children—and adults as well—were becoming less flexible, less strong—in short, less physically fit than their forefathers had been, and that they were worse off as a result.

The controversy spilled over into the press, and an article that I wrote for the *New York State Journal of Medicine* was picked up in a magazine published by the Amateur Athletic Association, and this came to the attention of a former athletic great, John B. Kelly. At the time he was best known to the public for being the father of Grace Kelly, but he had twice won Olympic gold medals for rowing and had been an adviser on physical fitness to the late President Franklin D. Roosevelt. When it came to physical fitness, Kelly played no political favorites. He called the article to the attention of the then President, Dwight Eisenhower, whom Kelly knew to be concerned with the problem. President Eisenhower then held a special sports luncheon at the White House, and he invited me and one of my research assistants, Mrs. Ruth Hirschland, to attend.

When we delivered our report, President Eisenhower, as the press later remarked, was shocked. The President subsequently established the Council for Physical Fitness. The physical educators now became interested but, in trying to get away from the word "physical," succeeded in having the name changed to the Council for Youth Fitness, ignoring the point that underexercise threatens not only children but the entire adult population. Almost all of them regarded the idea of formal exercise as unpalatable. Instead, they suggested various sports and games as an alternative. This sounds very well, but, as I point out in Chapter 7, some sports are better than others for physical conditioning and some sports may even be harmful. Sports were not and are not the answer. The answer was and is basic exercise programs geared to the correction of muscular deficiencies and development of good hearts and lungs.

At the time I simply did not realize that many physical educators had such an ingrained dislike of exercise. I found this out in 1957, when I attended a meeting with a number of physical educators. It was a very friendly session. After a few minutes we got down to the main problem. I asked, "Why are you against exercise?"

"We can't use exercises," one physical educator said.

"Why not?" I asked.

He smiled. "Very simple," he said. "Twenty-five years ago we gave exercises to school children. And as far as I'm concerned, that's enough. We were looked down on as the boobs of the school system. We had no status at all. So we changed our emphasis. Now who are we? Well, we're not the boobs we used to be. Now we're respected members of the academic community. We're educators, physical educators if you wish. We're not 'exercise teachers' any more. We're educators, coaches, and administrators. You want to know the truth? Exercise is finished! It's passé; it's out of date. You want us to turn back the clock. Well, I'm telling you, Doctor, we don't care what your findings show, we're not going back to the old days. We've worked hard to get where we are, and we're going to stay there."

Well, at least this was an honest answer. In the same way, the Council for *Youth* Fitness became increasingly bogged down in talk. At council meetings there was no point in bringing up exercise. Instead the physical educators discussed different forms of "fitness," mental fitness, moral fitness, youth fitness, psychological fitness, and so on.

The situation got worse. Even physicians did their best to avoid the problem. I remember that at a yearly council meeting I made the elementary proposal to a group of physicians that we collect all the medical literature relating to the merits or demerits of physical activity as a cause of disease. I couldn't even find one physician to second the motion, but another motion—that there was no such thing as any standard for physical fitness—was quickly made, seconded, and passed! The only dissenting vote was mine. I protested. Medicine had all sorts of standards, I said. There was a standard for blood pressure. There was a standard for blood count, pulse rate, blood sugar, and body temperature. But all this was pooh-poohed. Finally I said, with some irony, "All right, I hereby make the motion that a twelve-year-old child should be able to run ten steps without collapsing." I had no sooner said this than a pediatrician jumped up and said, in all seriousness, "Yes, but that is about as far as I would go on this motion."

When John F. Kennedy was elected President, he renewed interest in physical fitness, and he went right to the heart of the problem. He announced his concern in two articles he wrote for *Sports Illustrated.* In 1960 the late President reviewed the shocking results of the Kraus-Weber tests administered to youngsters in both America and Europe, and in 1962 he wrote in *Sports Illustrated* that a survey personally ordered by him revealed "that more than 10 million of our 40 million school children are unable to pass a test which measures only the minimum level of fitness, while almost 20 million would be unable to meet the standards set by a more comprehensive test of physical strength and skills.

"These figures," President Kennedy continued, "indicate the vast dimensions of a national problem which should be of deep concern to us all. It is paradoxical that the very economic progress, the technological advance and scientific breakthroughs which have, in part, been the result of our national vigor have also contributed to the draining of that vigor. Technology and automation have eliminated many of those physical exertions which were once a normal part of the working day. New forms of transportation have made it unnecessary to walk to school or to the office or the corner store. New forms of entertainment have consumed much of the time which was once used for sports and games.

"No one can deny the enormous benefits which these developments have brought—the reduction of drudgery and tedious tasks, the opportunity for greater leisure, the increased access to intellectual stimulation and quality entertainment. But at the same time we must not allow these advances to become the instruments of the decline of our national vitality and health. We cannot permit the loss

51

of that physical vigor which has helped nourish our growth and which is essential if we are to carry forward the complex and demanding tasks which are vital to our strength and progress."

Before his tragic death President Kennedy said that he intended to take a new look at the fitness program. He was well aware of the fact that little had been done to meet the problem.

Meanwhile other physicians took great interest in the problem, among them Dr. Paul Dudley White, the heart specialist, Dr. Wilhelm Raab, director of the Cardiovascular Research Unit at the University of Vermont College of Medicine, and Dr. Hans Selye of McGill University, who has done pioneering work in stress. Their research and experience strongly buttress the data that my associates and I have collected showing that lack of exercise combined with constant irritation produces an imbalance, a sickness in our emotional and physical functions.

As research piles up, the climate is gradually changing. Many physicians are now beginning to look upon exercise with favor, though there are still some diehards. After Dr. Kenneth Lane published a fine paper, "Role of Pediatricians in Physical Fitness of Youth," in a 1959 issue of the *Journal of the American Medical Association,* there were only ridiculing letters to the editor.

Still acceptance comes, however slowly. In 1964 the American Medical Association published a pamphlet on physical fitness. It notes, among other things, that physical activity is good protection against back pain caused by sedentary living, a helpful way of controlling weight, and a preventive of degenerative disease. The AMA pamphlet mentions that "diseases of the heart and blood vessels, diabetes, and arthritis strike the obese more often and more seriously than they strike those of desirable weight." The pamphlet further states that exercise may help relieve tension. Two pamphlets, *Vim* and *Vigor,* recently issued by the President's Council for Physical Fitness, also proclaim that exercise will make youngsters "radiate confidence" and allow them to win friends.

The fact is, however, that exercise cannot be made palatable on the grounds that it will help you glow with charm and grace. The blunt fact is that exercise, properly done, will help you prevent the onslaught of disease. Back pain is only one of the diseases that afflict the underexercised, and as I discuss back pain you should bear in mind that it is representative of many troubles that may come either to you or your children. If you or they are underexercised, you can start now to correct this condition, this sickness. It is not easy. It needs daily attention. But it is well worth it. Right now you accept as normal the overweight man of twenty-five or thirty who cannot run up two flights of stairs without huffing and puffing. You accept the fact—you even expect—that a businessman is tense and nervous and has high blood pressure, bad back, or ulcers. All too many doctors advise a forty-year-old who plays tennis to slow down and "act your age." Friends tell you that overweight, tension, muscular weakness, and occasional painful back are "normal." Nothing could be further from the truth.

CHAPTER 3

The Importance of the
Muscles and the Spine

IN ONE WAY or another most of us are status conscious, but when it comes to status, muscles do not rank. They are one of the most important parts of your body, but they are the least respected. This attitude is even reflected in popular speech. You will praise the brain or heart, but you have no respect at all for muscles. You speak in complimentary terms of a person when you say, "He's brainy," "She's got a brain," "She's got heart," or "He's a hearty fellow." But what do you say about muscles? You speak of them with contempt: "He's all muscle," "He's muscle-bound," "He's a muscle man," "Muscle Beach," and "He's muscling in on us."

Few physical educators show much respect for muscles either. Instead of seeing to it that youngsters grow up with strong and flexible muscles, too many of them think only of coaching winning teams or of becoming administrators.

Medical students are not instructed in therapeutic exercise or muscle evaluation. When you go for a thorough checkup, you are given an electrocardiogram, your blood pressure and pulse rate are taken, your nervous system, eyes and ears are examined, your blood and urine are analyzed, and your heart and lungs are examined. X-rays are taken of whatever body area is suspected of being diseased or injured. This is as it should be. But are your muscles examined for strength and flexibility? Very rarely. If tests are given, they gauge neurological deficiencies. Tests to detect whether your muscles can manage your body weight are uncommon, and so is appraisal of flexibility and muscle tension. Yet your muscles have a tremendous effect on your over-all health. Muscles are not only important and vital in themselves, but they exert great influence, for better or worse, on your metabolism and emotional life. Their use keeps your cardiovascular system in good shape. If you don't use your muscles sufficiently in running or other strenuous activities, your heart does not get the stimuli it needs to keep strong and healthy.

Your muscles do countless things for you. When you walk, you use your muscles. When you work with your hands, you use your muscles. When you move your back, you use your muscles. Your muscles, moreover, are your only means of communication with the outer world; they are irreplaceable organs of expression. When you show your thoughts and feelings by facial movements, when you talk, when you write, when you dance, you use your muscles. You must use them constantly to show what you feel and think. This applies to the abstract thinker as much as the day laborer. The thinker who is afflicted with back pain, stiff neck, or tension headache simply cannot function in top shape.

Besides allowing you to move and to express your thoughts, your muscles are the only organs which permit you to exert your will. In fact, you can use your muscles to train your will. For thousands of years some religions have deemed training of the body the first step toward disciplining the mind and the spirit. It is no wonder that symbolic movement and posture are an integral part of worship.

Use of your muscles affects your metabolism. If you exercise sufficiently, you will set up a natural balance against overweight. Until only a few decades ago most people had to work hard physically for their food. Their muscles and organs used up what they ate. In addition to regulating weight and metabolism, the heavy labor done by the muscles kept the heart and blood vessels in good condition. There is no denying that the death rate was higher in the "good old days," but the reason that we live longer now than people did in the seventeenth or eighteenth centuries is due largely to preventive medicine's victories over most types of contagious diseases, to antibiotics, sewage disposal, and milk control. As a matter of fact, the upsurge of longevity has come to a halt. In 1964 the U.S. Public Health Service reported that American life expectancy is on the decrease.

Yes, people now live longer than their ancestors did, but how many people really feel vibrant and alive? The answer, as I check our clinical records, is all too few.

Your muscles are only as good as you make them. When

you do not use the muscles of your body properly, they suffer and so do you. Neglect or abuse the muscles that keep your body erect, and you are bound to get back pain, stiff neck, or tension headache. When muscles are weak through lack of exercise and tense because of irritation, they cannot do their share of keeping the body erect and too much strain falls on the bones and ligaments of your spine. Let us take a look at the spine and the muscles involved in its function.

Your spine runs from your head to your buttocks. It consists, in order, of seven cervical or neck vertebrae, then twelve dorsal vertebrae in the middle back, then five lumbar vertebrae in the so-called small of the back and, finally, the sacrum, a bone of roughly triangular shape that connects the spinal column with the pelvis. The vertebrae, the bony parts of the spine, are not directly linked to one another but are separated by ligamentous rings with a soft inner part rather like a jelly doughnut. These rings are known as discs, and they are notorious as a source of serious back trouble. Fortunately "slipped" discs are not quite as common as you might think. As you will see in Chapter 5, many persons who think they are suffering from disc trouble actually are victims of muscle strain in the back, and this condition can be corrected through exercise instead of surgery.

Besides the discs, there are strong ligaments joining the vertebral bodies with one another and with the sacrum. On the back part of each vertebra is a bony ring. This holds the spinal cord. The center of this cord consists of nerve cells. Surrounding it are large cables of nerve-fibers that ultimately join the lower and upper part of the brain. From there smaller nerve cables branch out into all parts of the body. These are the nerve cables that transmit all sensations to us. They help conduct reflexes, and they contain all the connections to the muscles. These nerves, traveling through their cable links, transmit orders from the brain and the spinal cord that make muscles move and contract.

The spinal column is formed in the shape of a gentle "S." The ligaments and discs together make the spinal column an elastic structure. But in order to function correctly—and in order to offset sudden blows or continuous strain—the spinal column needs help. This help is given by the trunk muscles. All of them, not only the back muscles, but stomach muscles and hip flexors as well as hip extensors, support the spinal column. They combine to keep it erect. They allow the column to move. They protect the column by acting as an outer guard. If your muscles are really in good condition, they can even offset damage to the spinal column itself. As a case in point I will cite the story of a friend of mine, a mountain climber. I'll call him Alex. For years he has spent all his free time in the mountains. He regularly spent his weekends climbing the cliffs of the Shawangunk Mountains near New York City. He is in superb condition.

One Monday morning Alex unexpectedly showed up at our clinic. "What are you doing here?" I asked.

"Guess what!" he said, with a big smile. "I have a bad back."

I couldn't believe it. Furthermore, he was smiling about it.

Alex sat down painfully and told me what happened. "I went climbing yesterday, as usual," he said. "But this time I found no partner and foolishly decided to climb alone. I went up the southern 'pillar' and enjoyed the rock and the sun and being alone. Just when I was ready to pull myself up to the second belay place my right hand slipped and I fell. Down I went, bouncing off the rock a couple of times. Anyway, I came to a stop after some fifty feet straight down. I was lucky that my fall was broken by a bush and I landed on a wide ledge. I was knocked unconscious, and when I came to, I thought I was dead. But I wasn't. I felt for broken bones, but I couldn't feel any. I got up carefully. I ached all over, but the pain in the back was the worst. I'm still quite beaten up but not badly enough to go to the hospital. I just want to find out whether I have broken anything in my back."

We examined his back. Alex had a large swelling, a hematoma, covering the back from his buttocks to his shoulders. We took X-rays of the spine and couldn't believe it. There was no injury at all, and except for minor cuts and a slightly sprained ankle, the swelling on his back was his only serious injury. We drained the blood from the swelling. Three days later we did so again. A week afterward the back was black and blue, but the only pain Alex felt was in his sprained ankle. His strong and resilient back muscles had helped shield his spine from severe damage.

Besides strong and resilient back muscles, strong stomach

59

muscles and hip flexors are essential for the avoidance of back pain. When people complain of back pain, they invariably blame the back muscles. The pain is in the low back, to be sure, but the pain may be there because the stomach muscles or the hip flexors are weak. The muscles are weak because they are the most inactive ones in a sedentary life. Say you spend most of the day sitting down. When you sit, you still have to keep your back muscles active in order to avoid toppling over. At the same time you let your stomach muscles go slack, and your hip flexors are more or less inactive as well. This is as it should be, but if you do a lot of sitting and no exercise, these muscles are bound to become weak. And when they become weak, they impose a severe strain on the back muscles, and the back muscles simply are not up to carrying this strain of keeping your spine erect.

Keep this up consistently, add nervous irritation to your sedentary life, and the back muscles will get tense and stiff. Finally, when they are unable to stand the strain, they will rebel by going into spasm and causing pain. Weakness and tension often combine to produce pain, but tension does not necessarily have to be the result of emotional disturbance. The normal tension of work, especially of work done in a cramped position, may be enough to produce acute muscular tension that results in pain.

We had a good illustration of this three years ago. The patient was Dr. D., a psychiatrist in his middle fifties. Dr. D. was at the top of his profession, and his profession called for him to be sitting down all day. As a youngster he had been bookish and had done little exercise. When he became an analyst, he stopped doing what little exercise he had done. As a matter of fact, I figured that Dr. D. had spent close to thirty years just sitting down. For the last two years, he said, he had suffered back pain on and off. Examination revealed that his back was stiff. It was especially stiff on the left side. "That's the side to which I turn to face my patients," he said. I suggested that he change his seating arrangements. The examination also disclosed that Dr. D. had very weak stomach muscles. But one thing really struck me about Dr. D. He was completely relaxed otherwise. He was weak, but he had no trace of anxiety or mental tension. He was, in fact, so relaxed that when I had finished the examination, I said to him, "I hope you will excuse me for being personal, but you're rather unusual. You are one of the few patients I have seen who is really serene."

He smiled and said, "Yes, I guess I am. I'm very happily married, and my wife and I have raised good and useful children. I myself was brought up in a very devout home, and I was told as a boy that every human being has at least one good side and that he should be loved for that good side. I believe that, and I've always been very happy, both in my family life and in my work."

Dr. D. was an ideal patient. Since he had no emotional source of tension, he managed to deal with his working tension by frequently changing his position at work. He interrupted his day as often as possible by lying down and actively relaxing. He learned how to do this very quickly. For several months he came in and was treated by a therapist who administered exercises that limbered and stretched his back and leg muscles and strengthened his abdominal muscles. Dr. D. cannot fit sports or outdoor activities in his pattern of living. But he avoids back pain by continuing his exercises regularly at home and moving around in the office.

In order to produce strength, a muscle shortens and tightens. It becomes tense, and it performs whatever task you want it to do, whether it be lifting a pencil, moving your legs, or turning your head. After the muscle has performed the task, it normally returns to its initial length and goes into a state of relaxation. It stops being tense; other muscles take over, become tense, do their job, and in turn let go and return to a state of relaxation. It is this flowing rhythm of tensing and relaxing muscles that makes for smooth movement.

The more you use a muscle, the stronger it will become. Your stomach muscles and hip flexors, for example, are mainly developed by running and lifting. If you do little running and lifting, these muscles will not develop. They will be weak and will impose an unnatural strain upon the back muscles, as was the case with Dr. D. Luckily for him, he had no emotional tension to compound the problem. But he was a rarity. Most persons are tied in knots with tension.

Tension prohibits muscular relaxation. A muscle must relax. Relaxing is a part of its function. If a muscle fails to relax, it stays tight. It loses its stretch, its suppleness, its give. Over a period of time it becomes permanently shortened. When this happens, the muscle loses most of its ability to release tension. If you have tense and shortened muscles, you are susceptible to all sorts of "tension syn-

62

drome"—back pain, stiff neck, or headache—because your muscles never have the chance to let go or relax, and neither do you.

Your muscles can be trained, if you take the trouble to train them properly. They can become strong and relaxed through purposeful exercise, or they can become shortened and tense from lack of exercise and over-irritation. Like mischievous children, muscles are more inclined to stick to bad habits than persist in good ones. How they behave is up to you. Overtensing and shortening of your muscles are very bad habits, and once acquired, they may be hard to break. You can see this around you all the time. Look at people you know are tense. How do they move their bodies? Certainly not smoothly. Their body movements are not fluid or rhythmic but jerky and stiff. They freeze themselves into a position, whether they are sitting in a chair, standing, or driving a car. They force their muscles into a steady alert reaction. Their muscles, already under tension, are forced to become even more tense. The muscles of the neck, shoulder girdle, and back are particularly tense, and they become the prime target areas for even more tension.

Look at your friend who is usually tense. Watch him at the wheel of a car when you're with him. It's the morning rush hour, and he is late for the office. Whenever a horn blows behind him or he misses a green light or a car cuts in front, you can almost see his shoulder muscles tense with each irritation. This happens to you, too, and the irritations keep up all day long. Each time you are irritated the muscles become tense. As the irritations keep up, the muscles keep tensing, and they never get the chance to respond normally and relax.

Irritations come from all over. There are external irritations, such as traffic jams, the ringing of the telephone, a sudden loud noise, an unexpected slap on the back, a shout from your children. These are just samples of hundreds that occur every day. Then there are internal irritations; just thinking about them can make your muscles tense. You do not like your job; a member of the family is desperately ill; your sexual relations are a problem. All these internal irritations can make your muscles extremely tense, tense to the point of inducing muscle spasm and pain. Sexual difficulties, for instance, can have a devastating effect. Take, for example, the case of Harry G.

Mr. G. was an accountant in his late thirties. Five years previous to treatment he had been married. He saw us on the recommendation of his psychiatrist. Mr. G. had back pain. He was extremely tense. He was also nearly impotent, which was why he had been seeing the psychiatrist. Three months after his honeymoon he strained his back while trying to change a flat tire. Up to then sexual relations had not been completely satisfactory; after he hurt his back muscles he came to dread intercourse because it produced pain. In time he actually equated intercourse with pain while simultaneously he began to brood about his apparent lack of masculinity. Muscular pain and emotional tension like this can really wreck a person. Back pain and his feeling of inferiority became part of a continuous vicious cycle that almost destroyed Harry G. emotionally and physically.

While the psychiatrist worked on Mr. G.'s mind, we

worked on his back. Slowly but gradually his back began to improve. Slowly but gradually the psychiatrist was able to allay his fears. It took almost a year before Mr. G. began to show signs of definite improvement. When the vicious circle was broken, his life returned to normal.

In the last two decades medicine has started to pay a great deal of attention to emotional stress and tension. Psychiatric treatment is often advised. It is only in recent years, however, that some doctors, including psychiatrists, have begun to realize that tension pain may be caused by both mental *and* physical factors. Unfortunately too few persons know how to move their muscles and their bodies, much less control their emotions. Instead of mastering their emotions, they have let emotion master them, unaware that emotions are the wellsprings of muscle tension. Since many persons lack both emotion and physical discipline, their lives become subject to moods, emotional storms, anxieties, and hostilities. These factors only make muscle tension all the worse and they are an important source of hypokinetic disease.

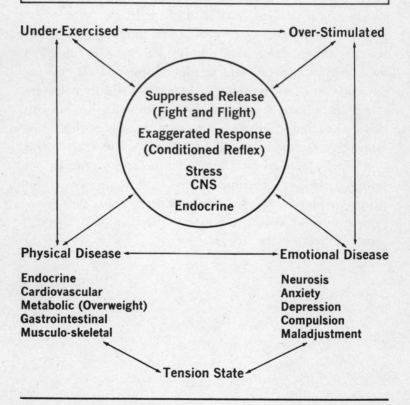

MECHANIZED, URBANIZED, UNBALANCED INDIVIDUAL

Over-Rested   Over-Fed   Over-Stimulated

Over-Protected   Under-Exercised   Under-Released

Under-Disciplined

Under-Exercised ←——————→ **Over-Stimulated**

Suppressed Release
(Fight and Flight)

Exaggerated Response
(Conditioned Reflex)

Stress
CNS

Endocrine

Physical Disease ←——————→ **Emotional Disease**

Endocrine   Neurosis
Cardiovascular   Anxiety
Metabolic (Overweight)   Depression
Gastrointestinal   Compulsion
Musculo-skeletal   Maladjustment

Tension State

(Documented in "Hypokinetic Disease" by H. Kraus and W. Raab, Charles C Thomas, Publisher.)

CHAPTER 4

Fight or Flight:
Why Tension Builds

A FEW THOUSAND years ago, a short time in the history of a species, man lived in caves. He led the life of a brute animal. He was physically involved in the struggle for existence. So were his wife and children. Like all animals, their bodies were endowed with an amazingly complex and efficient preparation for action. In an instant their bodies were ready to fight or to flee. In either case they responded with a physical action. They either fought or they fled.

Civilized man—and civilized woman—has the same physiological structure. When you are faced with a stressful situation, your body prepares to act. But unlike your ancestors, you neither fight nor flee. The rules of civilized society prevent this, and usually you do nothing but sit and seethe. This constant suppression of a natural physical response puts an unnatural strain on your system.

Here is a typical case. Angela J. was a slim brunette secretary in her late twenties. Her posture was bad, her neck stiff. She was as tense as any girl who ever came to our clinic.

"For the past three years," she said, "I have had pain, both in my neck and in the back of my shoulders. No matter what I do, the pain just will not go away.

"I first got a pain in the neck when I went to work for the Blank Company"—and here Angela named a large corporation—"three years ago. I'm a secretary. There's an awful lot of work to do; we're almost always shorthanded, and I would have quit, but I have friends there. A month after I started work I got a stiff neck. I had it a couple of days. I remember thinking that I had caught it working near a new air conditioner. It went away. But about a month after that I had to fill in for another girl and I got a stiff neck again. This time there was no air conditioner nearby. I tried to do different things for the pain, like putting hot packs on it, but I just couldn't seem to loosen it up.

"After I went back to my regular boss I was all right for a little while. Then I started getting pain between my shoulder blades. First it was at the end of the day, then at lunch. Now it starts in the morning.

"Last month it started to get worse. I got the pain between the shoulders before I even went to work. Yesterday was the worst day I've ever had. My boss was off on a trip, but he phoned long distance and told me he wanted to change some letters he had dictated the day before. I had just finished typing them up, and I was furious. I took the new dictation down on the phone, and I started to retype the letters. I was halfway through the first one when the pain simply became too much to take. I got up and walked away from the typewriter and tried to relax. I couldn't. So I sat down again and started to type. But I simply could not continue. My neck felt locked, and in between my shoulder blades it felt as though my muscles were in knots. I had to stop work. I feel hopeless."

I assured Angela that she need not feel hopeless, and I asked her what she thought prompted the pain. She guessed it was her work, but then she dismissed this by saying that was "only in her head."

I agreed that the pain was started by what was in her head. I told her that her muscles reacted to the constant mental irritations and frustrations of the job by getting ready to strike out or run away. Since Angela neither ran away nor struck out, since she never fulfilled "the fight or flight response," her muscles remained tense, in a state of constant readiness. Inasmuch as this had happened day after day after day over three years, her muscle tension had finally reached the state where it became painful. At first she had felt the pain at the end of a long day. Then, as the tension started to accumulate, it took less and less irritation to produce the pain. The phone call from her boss had brought her pain to a climax.

"In short," I told Angela, "you undergo rage without hitting, and fear without fleeing. Instead of resolving the situation, you stay at your work, hunching your shoulders and seething inwardly. Instead of fighting or fleeing, you seethe. Your neck and shoulder muscles haven't relaxed in three years. Now they have gotten so tense that they rebelled by going into spasm."

I told Angela to stay away from work for a week while she began treatment. It was an involved case, requiring physical therapy to relieve her muscle spasm and medication to relieve pain and to calm her nerves. She then needed exercises to limber her neck and shoulder muscles, and she had to learn exercises that would relax her.

Two weeks passed before Angela could return to her job. Even then she still required treatment. Three weeks after returning to work her neck and back muscles began to become painful again. This time I suggested that she look around for another job where working conditions were easier, where there would be little if no tension. After all, I told her, a good secretary can always get another job, and she would still have her friends. Angela did as suggested and had no trouble at all in getting another position with fewer irritating demands. Since then she has kept up her exercise program, and she has been doing well. Her neck and shoulders remain sensitive to strain and irritation, but Angela now recognizes the warning signs of "fight or flight" and knows how to handle them.

Failure to respond with a physical action to fight or flight is the main cause of tension. It has become particularly important as more and more people lead lives without exercise. Underexercised muscles never get a chance to get rid of tension.

What happens to you physiologically when you are challenged or irritated? A number of things: adrenalin pours into your system; your heart beats faster; you breathe quicker; your blood pressure rises, and your muscles tense. In the days when men and women led primitive lives, they completed this response either by fighting or running away.

But what do you do? You do nothing except seethe. Your muscles, your mind, your heart, and your organs all prepare to act, but you do nothing. You may want to fight, you may wish to flee, but modern civilization prevents you from carrying out your natural impulses. When the boss tell you off, you have to "grin and bear it," and you only get more tense. Then there are occasions when you cannot respond physically even should you wish to do so. You cannot throw the telephone at the pest on the other end of the line. You cannot punch the insane driver doing seventy miles an hour who just missed hitting you with his car. In such situations you neither fight nor flee. Instead, you do as you usually do; you seethe. This happens to you all the time, and this constant suppression of physical response puts a strain on the muscles that tense and want to react.

Think of all the times during the day when your body gets ready to respond to a challenge or an irritation. Then think of all the times you do absolutely nothing. All this has an appalling effect on your ready-to-respond system, especially when the pattern is repeated day in and day out, month after month, year after year. Now I am not talking about lurid or dramatic situations where you are called upon to defend your life or your honor. I am talking about the flood of daily irritations that bedevil and bother you.

You don't have to be facing a mugger with a knife to have your system sound battle stations. Your system actually prepares for action when the phone rings, when someone shouts at you, when you hear a sudden noise, when you are interrupted at work, when you hear your child fall down and burst loudly into tears. Your whole being gets set to respond, to fight or to flee. Your muscles suddenly tense up. They get ready to act. So does your heart, your blood vessels, your glands, and your mind. But you do nothing. All day long the irritations mount up, making your muscles tense and putting your mind in a state of anxiety and irritation. But you race your engines without ever going anywhere. As sure as anything, this is almost guaranteed to trigger back pain, a stiff neck, or a thudding tension headache. And this may be only one of many other adverse results. The same unreleased strain, if repeated often, may cause high blood pressure, ulcers, or heart disease. Surely it will upset you emotionally and make you "nervous."

Medicine owes its knowledge of the fight or flight response to a great researcher, the late physiologist, Walter B. Cannon of Harvard. Cannon wanted to know what happened to man when he underwent fear or rage, and he began by experimenting on animals. What happened to laboratory animals when they were irritated? Cannon studied their reactions. The animals tensed their muscles. They increased their heartbeats, and blood pressure rose quickly. Adrenalin was released into the blood stream and raised the blood sugar to provide emergency rations for the muscle, and sugar spilled into the urine. In the wild this preparation for action is essential. The animal reacts physically to the irritation. It fights or it flees. Then afterward the muscles relax, blood pressure drops, the heartbeat slows, and breathing becomes normal.

A cat is a perfect example of this. When a cat is not disturbed, it is perfectly at ease. Every muscle is supple and relaxed. Yet when the cat becomes irritated or angered, you can watch it become tense before your eyes. It spits, hisses; it arches its back as it prepares to fight or to flee. When the irritation reaches a certain point, the cat either attacks or runs away. In either case it carries out a physical response. The cat does not sit and stew like you do. It responds physically, and after it does it returns to its state of ease and relaxation.

Cannon went on further with his research. He found his results confirmed in human beings. For example, he and a colleague checked the urine of twenty-five Harvard football players after a Yale game. Sugar was found in the urine of twelve excited players, five of them substitutes who sat on the bench throughout. An excited spectator examined also had sugar in his urine.

Besides Cannon's pioneering research, various other investigators have conducted experiments on muscle tension. A German physiologist, Tiegel, did research showing that repeated tensing of a muscle results in a definite loss of length. The muscle shrinks, so to speak, and when suddenly you are required to stretch it, it cannot do the job and it reacts by going into spasm or, even worse, tearing. A pair of English physicians, Peter Sainsbury and T. G. Gibson, did interesting experiments on tension pain. They examined a number of people who complained of habitual

73

tension headache or muscle pain. They used a device to measure action currents in the muscles. When a muscle contracts it produces weak electric currents; the intensity of the currents is in proportion to the degree of muscle contraction. One set of electrodes was attached to the muscle or muscles producing the pain—the "target" area—and another set was affixed to "normal" muscles that did not produce pain. Then Sainsbury and Gibson put the subjects through an interview deliberately designed to bring about tension. As the interview proceeded, Sainsbury and Gibson discovered that the normal muscles started to tense but relaxed quickly afterward. The muscles that produced pain, however, not only started to tense during the interview but tensed even more afterward, bringing about pain at the peak of contraction.

There are definite "target areas" of muscle tension in tension headache; they are the occipital muscles running up the back of the head and the frontalis muscles in the forehead. Sometimes you can feel the tight occipital muscles if you have a very bad headache. Put your fingers behind your head midway between the upper part of your ears and the back of the skull, and you may feel your muscles tighten. The target areas for painful or stiff necks are the neck muscles and the trapezius muscles, which cover your shoulder blades, and the rhomboid muscles which are beneath the trapezius. The muscles of the lower back are prime target areas. Less frequently target areas are found in the legs, thighs, arms, or any place where muscles are continually subjected to tension without release and relaxation.

Sometimes you can be bothered by one particular irritation and not realize it. This reminds me of a Mrs. M., a forty-year-old career woman who came to have a stiff neck treated. She carried her neck twisted to the right side and was quite uncomfortable. We were able to limber it up somewhat on her initial visit. Mrs. M. had a very responsible job with a publishing company. After loosening her neck, I started talking about her tension and the need to find its source to minimize it. I had no idea as to what specific irritation was triggering her stiff neck until she glanced at her wrist watch and said, "This is all very interesting, but I must be back at the office at three to dictate to my secretary." As soon as she said the word "secretary," her neck at once twisted to the right.

"Don't be in such a hurry, Mrs. M.," I said. "I have an idea of what's wrong."

Mrs. M. stayed. It turned out that she could not stand her secretary. The girl was pleasant enough but inefficient to an extreme. Mrs. M. had put up with her for two years. She had thought many times of firing her, but when she remembered her own beginnings in business and the difficult time she had had, she always relented.

When Mrs. M. returned a week later, her neck was again stiff. I suggested that she change secretaries. Mrs. M. wouldn't hear of it, but when the neck pain persisted for a month, she finally resolved to transfer the girl. The girl literally was a pain in the neck.

CHAPTER 5

Why We Get
Sick Backs

ORGANIC DISEASE causes only a small percentage of back pain. X-rays sometimes show "osteoarthritic" changes of the vertebrae, but these do not often cause pain. Rheumatoid arthritis, a much more serious ailment, causes pain and stiffness, but it is relatively rare. Other pathologies, such as malignancies and tuberculosis of the spine, are still more unusual. Even "disc" trouble is not as common as one might think. The same is true of mechanically unstable spine caused by congenital malformation or injury. In short, if you suffer from back pain, the chances are that your condition is caused, not by organic disease, but by muscles that are weak or tense or both.

A number of medical researchers have found this to be the case. Dr. Weber and I found this out for ourselves at the special back-pain clinic organized at Columbia-Presbyterian Hospital. More than 80 per cent of the patients who complained of back pain were found to be suffering from muscular deficiencies, while less than 20 per cent had pathological disorders. Drs. Barbara Stimson and Sawnie Gaston arrived at a similar figure. All of us were able to arrive at this conclusion because the patients treated at the clinic were thoroughly examined by a team of physicians specializing in all sorts of fields. In addition, every patient was given X-rays, and laboratory analyses were made of his blood and urine. In short, nothing was left unexamined in the quest to find the reasons for complaints of back pain.

The muscularly deficient back-pain sufferers would have been considered "healthy," except for the fact that they had pain. Then when they took the six K-W tests, they all failed one or more. They simply did not have the necessary muscle strength to manage their own body weight and/or they lacked the muscular flexibility required for their own size. When given prescribed exercises, the majority improved. A follow-up more than a decade later showed that as long as these patients did their exercises every day they had relief from pain and their muscles were strong and resilient.

Many of these patients had localized and exquisitely tender spots which we could feel in their muscles. These spots are called "trigger points." They were first extensively described by a German orthopedic surgeon, Max Lange, more than fifty years ago and then by another well-known specialist, Arthur Steindler, in this country. In recent years many other physicians have written about trigger points. Among them are Dr. Janet Travell and lately Drs.

Alois Brugger and Duri Gross of Zurich University, who have written an excellent monograph on the subject.

Trigger points occur in different parts of the body, but they are especially frequent in neck, shoulders, upper and lower backs, and hip muscles. They can be caused by constant or acute strain of the muscles or by muscle spasm. They are, in a sense, rather like scar tissue of muscles. Trigger points are very painful, and they can literally trigger pain by provoking muscle tension, spasm, or contracture. Trigger points usually appear in your muscles if you let minor episodes of back pain go untreated, and then, once the trigger points have formed, the episodes of pain will increase, both in intensity and frequency.

When we examine a patient with chronic back pain caused by weakness or tension, we feel the muscles gently with our fingers to see if there are trigger points. If there are none, exercise therapy can start once pain subsides, usually after about a week. We use ethyl chloride spray and other physical therapy to help relieve the pain.

If a patient has trigger points, we mark the locations on the skin. Then we inject each trigger point with procaine. This kills the pain, but more important, both the needling and the injected fluid itself break up the trigger point through the force of hydraulic pressure. Once the trigger points have been injected and eliminated by subsequent treatment, the patient can embark on an exercise program.

On occasion a physician may find another kind of tenderness when he gently rolls a patient's skin between his fingers. If the skin itself is very sensitive to the touch, it is known as "fibrositis." It responds well to pinching massage if carried out regularly for weeks, sometimes months.

Some patients are quite disappointed when they learn that their pain is caused by trigger points. They had expected "slipped" discs, caused when the ligamentous disc covers tear or give so that the soft contents ooze out and press nerve roots. These patients find it difficult to accept the fact that their trouble is "only muscles." Some even feel "left out" with such an unglamorous problem because so many movie stars and celebrities seem to be suffering from discs.

Trigger points and discs can be confused. Confusion sets in because they can exhibit similar symptoms. Like discs, trigger points can prompt radiating pain in either the upper and lower back and down the back of the legs or arms as well. But here the similarities between trigger points and discs end. Trigger points do not cause reflex loss. Damaged discs can. Trigger points do not cause sensory loss, numbness, or weakness. Discs can.

Sometimes weak and stiff muscles, emotional tensions, endocrine imbalance, muscle tenderness, or skin tenderness all combine to cause pain and make a diagnosis difficult. You can understand how such a complicated condition may lead to a diagnosis of "disc trouble," even though there may be no real involvement of a disc. Occasionally these symptoms suggest at least impending disc lesion.

It has happened that some back-pain sufferers with trigger points have been incorrectly diagnosed as having disc trouble. This can be harmful, because from that moment on a patient, seeing surgery as a distinct possibility, is asked to "live with" the pain and to refrain from "excessive motion." So the patient, who is really troubled by trigger points, becomes more and more inactive and thus worse off. Occasional minor spurts of activity only serve to inflict greater pain on the patient's constantly deteriorating muscles and sensitive trigger points. The downward trend becomes difficult to reverse, and complications set in, prompted by the patient's anxieties, such as the fear of surgery, the fear of disability, the fear of losing his livelihood. When a patient has reached this desperate stage, he or she loses all sense of emotional and active well-being and becomes resigned to a life of physical inactivity instead of a life of activity and vigor. On occasion such a patient will finally undergo surgery to remedy the "disc trouble," and of course this only does more harm since the muscles are made even weaker and tenser by long confinement to a hospital bed. And yet there are some back-pain sufferers who hate to be told that they have muscularly deficient backs instead of disc trouble, because discs are glamorous!

Even in cases of disc trouble surgery is not necessarily called for. There are times, many times as a matter of fact, when exercises to retrain inadequate muscles can offset damage to the spinal column. This was true of a patient whom I'll call Mr. Jim C. Mr. C. was in his early forties, and when he came to the clinic with pain in his back and right leg, he had already been through two operations for spinal fusion and removal of a disc. Yet the pain persisted. We had no doubt that he did have disc trouble before, and we had little doubt that he did have disc trouble again.

But rather than force Mr. C. to undergo surgery yet again, we thought it would be worthwhile to try different treatment. Mr. C. readily agreed; he had little desire to spend more time in the hospital flat on his back.

First Mr. C. had to take a full month's leave of absence from his job as an executive in a large manufacturing firm. This eliminated tension at work which, incidentally, had been aggravated by Mr. C.'s poor postural habits in handling the telephone. We used the first month of treatment to deal with painful trigger points in Mr. C.'s back and hip. A gradual retraining program was also started. Rest at home, use of a surgical corset, and muscle relaxants were prescribed. Later when Mr. C. returned to work, he continued to come to the clinic for exercise sessions three times a week. He did exercises at home the other days.

It took more than six months for Mr. C.'s muscles to return to normal, and during that time he was slowly weaned from his corset. Even when he felt all right he had to return to the clinic for periodic checkups. In the beginning he suffered one or two mild setbacks when he stood too long and when he started playing golf prematurely.

Mr. C. now lives a normal life, but he has to continue to keep in good condition. His back remains his weak spot, reacting when he is under too much stress of any kind. He now knows the signs of trouble, however, and he has learned how to handle them.

Exercise may also be used for treatment of "mechanically unstable spine" caused by old fractures, worn-out joints of the vertebrae, and by forward sliding of the last (fifth) lumbar vertebra on the sacrum. In these cases, however, effectiveness of exercise is limited and surgery may be needed.

There are, of course, occasions when surgery is imperative. Once a very attractive young blonde in her late twenties, Miss Jane S., came to us for treatment. Six years before she had taken a trip to Europe. On the ship on the way back she tripped and fell down a ladder. Miss S. felt pain and stiffness in her back but did not see a physician. From then on she was never entirely free from backache. When we saw her, Miss S. seemed to be in good physical condition, but there was no doubt she was stiff and felt pain. X-rays were ordered. They disclosed an old fracture of the fourth lumbar vertebra. We recommended a spinal fusion, and it was performed successfully. A reconditioning period of exercise followed. Only occasional discomfort reminds her now of past injury.

We have seen how many factors—underexercise, tension, glandular imbalance, and severe injury—may cause back pain, but other factors—overweight, flat feet, unequal leg length, and poor seating or sleeping facilities—may play a part. All these factors create a situation which gradually may lead to backache, maybe starting at night after a long day, as fatigue pain, or discomfort and stiffness in the morning or after long periods of sitting as "jelling pain." Discomfort may gradually increase in degree and spread to your thighs or arms. Finally you reach the point where you are never comfortable. Often a sudden minor blow, a sudden twisting motion, sudden stooping, or lifting may set off an acute, sudden attack of pain that may force you to go to bed or even to the hospital. Even minimal injury will be sufficient to do this if you are in poor muscular condition and have had low-grade backache for some time.

In a healthy person whose back is protected by strong, resilient muscles it takes a much more serious injury to produce an attack of back pain. But the difference between injury to a healthy person and a deconditioned one goes further: the healthy person recovers much quicker under adequate care.

A case in point was Miss N., a dancer, who saw us two years after a second operation for disc trouble. After both operations she had felt fine—until she took up dancing again. Then severe pain forced her to give up performing. After the second operation she had tried several times to return to the stage only to be forced to give it up again. She thought about having a third operation. Examination revealed that Miss N. had extremely weak trunk muscles and stiff back and leg muscles. They were riddled with trigger points. Why? Because she had bravely tried to return to her demanding work without ever having gone through systematic reconditioning. It took several months of injections and exercise sessions to get her in good shape. She resumed her work and since then has missed few performances.

There are innumerable patients with similar experiences. Complete reconditioning after injury is a must for all physically active people. If they are properly reconditioned, they are not so likely to suffer again, no matter how physically demanding their work may be. Take the case of Dr. John L., a rugged country veterinarian. He was in his forties, and all his life he had been extremely active. In his spare time Dr. L. walked, ran, rode horseback, went hunting, fished, chopped wood, and played tennis. He was most vigorous physically. Even his job made physical demands upon him. He regularly went around the countryside shoeing horses, lifting sheep and hogs, and chasing cattle. One stormy night when Dr. L. was at home reading, the phone rang. It was a farmer who lived off in the hills ten miles away. The farmer said there was something wrong with his prize bull. Dr. L., like a family physician on call, set out at once in his car. He got to the farmer's place and, after the call was finished, said good night to the farmer and started home. It was still blowing hard outside. Two miles down the road from the farmer's house a huge ash tree had fallen across the road. Rather than drive back and trouble the farmer, Dr. L. decided he might as well chop the way free. He got an ax from the back of the car and started chopping. It took him about an hour to cut up the trunk so his car could get through. Then, feeling in good spirits, he decided to lift up one of the logs and throw it instead of rolling it to the side. When Dr. L. picked up the heavy log, he felt something twinge in his back. He dropped the log and rolled it to the side with his feet, got back in the car, and drove home.

Dr. L. had back pain for a week. He thought nothing more of it when it went away. But from then on the pain would return periodically, especially when he moved something heavy. After two years of on-and-off pain Dr. L. came into the clinic for treatment. He was perfectly healthy and had excellent muscles. The only thing was that he had a trigger point in the back muscles on his left side. We injected it with procaine and treated him for a few days. After that he learned some exercises to keep limbered. This treatment lasted only ten days. Now his outlook is good—he may never have any trouble again.

Whenever we treat back pain, we try to find its cause. A disc injury will require bed rest, maybe surgery. Fractures may need immobilization or surgery. Aside from these and other less frequent causes, we first treat "acute back strain" mainly by stopping muscle spasm. We use ethyl chloride spray, supported by electric muscle stimulation and gentle limbering motions given by a therapist. Others use applications of ice or hot packs. Whenever possible, gentle limbering performed at one-hour or half-hour intervals should be combined with rest to avoid unnecessary stiffening of the afflicted area. Muscle relaxants or pain-relieving medication may be given. Once the pain subsides, we start the patient on a prescribed exercise program.

There are cases—they are not common, but they occur from time to time—when exercise or surgery are of little or no use by themselves. For example, take the case of Mrs. Annette C. She was in her late forties and extremely emotional. She was close to being what she called "a complete wreck," and she looked it. Her hair was frowzy and her clothes sloppy. She was sent to us by her psychiatrist. Mrs. C. complained of severe back pain. From her medical record we knew that she was undergoing menopause. She had all the symptoms of chronic back pain, including very poor and stiff muscles. She came for treatment over a three-month period, and while her muscles improved, she did not. I knew from consulting with her psychiatrist that he was making no headway. We finally suggested that Mrs. C. visit an endocrinologist. She did, and the endocrinologist agreed that her menopause might help cause her emotional problems and recurring tension pain. He gave her medication, and Mrs. C.'s emotional tension and back pain subsided.

Similarly a Mr. Ronald A. came into the clinic complaining of muscle pain all over his body but especially in the back. He moved well enough, but he was putting on weight, his skin was dry, his hair was brittle. We sent him to an internist, who confirmed our suspicion that Mr. A. had a low thyroid function. Mr. A. remained under the observation of his internist and has been fine since his physician has kept him on adequate thyroid medication.

A patient named Richard M. complained that he woke up with stiff muscles in the morning. Mr. M. was in his early twenties, and like many young persons, he never had had a complete medical checkup. I insisted that he have one inasmuch as his stiffness seemed out of proportion to his age and general appearance. The checkup by an internist disclosed that Mr. M. was suffering from rheumatoid arthritis of the spine. Therapy and exercises were an important adjunct to his treatment, but his basic problem was the concern of his internist.

Such cases are not in the majority. Most back pain, stiff neck, or tension headache are due to a muscular imbalance, overstrain and underexercise. If you should suffer an attack of back pain at home or at work, lie down on a hard surface. A hard mattress over a board is best. The painful muscles should be covered with a hot pack composed of a towel dipped in boiling water and then wrapped in a dry towel. To avoid scalding, make sure that the wet towel has been wrung out completely. What really counts is not how long the towel stays hot on your back but the fact that it is hot to begin with. The sudden heat of a very hot towel shocks the muscles, and this helps to relieve the pain. Continue to rest on a hard surface until a physician arrives.

If you do not have back pain and yet cannot pass all six K-W tests, you still need help. You are leaving yourself not only exposed to muscle pain but, in the long run, to the other hypokinetic diseases as well: obesity, ulcers, diabetes, heart trouble, and emotional instability.

Fortunately this can be prevented or remedied. You will have to take stock of yourself. You can learn how to combat tension. You can learn how to exercise properly to correct any faults you have.

CHAPTER 6

Exercises
for Sick Backs

IF YOU HAVE FAILED one or more of the six
Kraus-Weber tests described in Chapter 1, you need help.
You are underexercised and/or overtensed, and this may
well be the breeding ground for future sickness. The K-W
tests are designed to test the key muscle groups in your
body, no matter what your age, height, or weight. These
tests are self-correlating. They do not judge you by some
outside arbitrary standard; they do not ask you to be as
strong as a coal miner or as lithe as an acrobat. Instead,
these tests simply reveal whether or not you have sufficient
muscular strength to move your own body weight and the
muscular flexibility to match your own size. By taking the
K-W tests, you will know for certain whether you are
muscularly below the minimum requirements for health-
ful living. You may have weak stomach muscles that need
strengthening; you may have stiff back muscles, or you

may find that you are tense. Then again you may have a combination of weaknesses. But once you know your deficiencies, you can do prescribed exercises designed to correct these specific difficulties. These are exercises with a purpose, to right what is wrong with you.

You may have been given exercises previously and they may not have helped. Do not let that discourage you. You may not have done the correct kind of exercise the right way for a long enough time. You might be able to decide this for yourself by answering the following questions: Have you been given a muscle test before exercises were prescribed? If not, the chances are you were not given the correct exercises. Were these exercises just given to you without detailed descriptions of how they were to be performed? If so, the chances are you didn't do them properly. Were you supposed to do all the exercises at once, or were you given a gradually increasing sequence? If you were given the whole program at once, the chances are it was not effective. Were you told to repeat each exercise many times, say five, ten, or more? If so, this may have been too much. Have you done your exercises every day, gradually increasing the number of minutes up to twenty or thirty minutes, slowly, relaxed, and consistently, for several months? If not, again, you may have missed the boat.

Giving a patient therapeutic exercise is a craft, even an art, and so is the prescribing of exercises. An exercise program should follow a rationale; it should be preceded by a thorough investigation of what has to be changed, and why, so as to give proper attention for your individual needs. An exercise prescription should be regarded as a potent medicine, which it is if properly given. You would not go to a drugstore with a prescription that simply said medicine or laxative. Instead, you would expect your prescription to be fully detailed as to what you were to get, how much, and when. The same thing is true for therapeutic exercise. You should get the proper type, in the proper dosage.

The exercises you will see in this chapter are not very spectacular or unusual. A number of them are prescribed by many physicians, by specialists in physical medicine and rehabilitation, and by therapists. You will select the exercises that fit your individual needs; you will do them the way they are prescribed, and you will build up your exercises gradually day by day until you have reached the full program. If you do your exercises properly, you will find them surprisingly effective. Bear in mind, however, that there is no easy way to accomplish improvement. There is no such thing as a fast five minutes a day to develop strong and flexible muscles. If you really wish to improve yourself, you will have to work. Think of an athlete training to run the mile in competition. He may be a fast runner, but before he can hit the four-minute mile and get into national and international competition, he has to work unceasingly and systematically for weeks and months, even years. When he has reached his peak, he will still have to continue training to remain in condition. Now you are not trying to break a record, but you are trying to get from below par to par, and that is often harder than trying to set a record.

Before going any further, I want to give you the basic ground rules for proper exercise:

1. *Check with your physician to make certain that you do not have an ailment that could be made worse by exercising now.* Do not start exercising if you have back pain or have had it in the past without making sure that your condition does not require medical care.

2. It is imperative that, once you start exercising, you keep at it every day. It is better not to start exercising at all unless you do so regularly. This is an important point, and it cannot be stressed enough. To be sure, there will be days when travel, important business, or emergencies will cut into your time, but don't go looking for excuses to avoid exercising. If you start and then stop an exercise program, you quickly lose what you have gained.

3. Avoid fatigue which might cause undue stiffness and soreness. Start with very gentle movements and gradually ease into your full program. If you are stiff and tense but strong, these exercises may seem "sissy stuff" to you, but you should still do them gradually. Do not try to accomplish everything in a short time. It is harder to learn how to relax, limber, and stretch than it is to develop strength.

4. Set aside a half hour a day for your daily exercises. Make that a "holy" half hour when you are not subjected to visitors, phone calls, or interferences or distractions of any kind. You owe this to yourself and your

own peace of mind. It is immaterial whether you do the exercises in the morning, afternoon, or evening, but do not do them immediately after a meal. Perhaps you will want to do them in the morning because you feel that they prepare you for the day. The only danger here is that there may be mornings when you are rushed, and you should not do the exercises if you feel it necessary to do them quickly. Never rush through them. If you have to leave early in the morning, do the exercises later in the day when you can make the time and have privacy.

    5. Never say that you are "too irritated" to do the exercises. The day that you feel too harried or put upon is the day you need the exercises most of all, particularly if you are exercising to release tension. A busy day will make you and your muscles tense, but if you do your exercises properly you will find the tension ebbing away. The tension that your muscles store up during a hectic day can be released through the exercises.

    6. Get in a relaxed state of mind for the exercises. If you follow instructions, you will learn how to do this. In your half hour of exercise put the cares of the world behind you, no matter how pressing or urgent they may seem to be. In this half hour nothing is more important than the job at hand. If a problem is particularly pressing or vexing, ask yourself, what will it matter fifty years from now? Live one day at a time. Exercise one session at a time. At first you will need only five to ten minutes for these sessions. They will gradually increase in time to approximately a half hour as you add exercises. Do not do a full program the first day or even the first week. Do only three or four of the exercises the first day. Never add more than one new exercise every two or three days—add them less often if the last exercise seems hard to do. All these exercises are planned in logical sequence. You start with a warm-up, say the first three exercises, reach a peak with the fourth, then work your way back, doing the first three exercises *in reverse order* so that what were the warm-up exercises end as the cool-off exercises. You always repeat your exercises in reverse order.

7. *Never do more than two or three of the same exercises in succession.* If your program is complete, you may want to go through it twice in one day, if you feel the need for extra work. Never do the exercises more frequently than that. Repetition will make you stiff, and chances are that lack of flexibility is one of your problems.

8. Your exercises must be performed slowly and smoothly. Do not do jerky movements, do not strain, do not "goose-step." Be sure you stop after each exercise and rest for a second before starting the next one. That means a pause between each exercise, not only each set of exercises.

9. Always start with the first six exercises, regardless of how you did on the K-W tests. If you are tense they will make you relax, and if you are weak they will give you a very mild warm-up. If you are strong but need relaxing and stretching, they are doubly important. If you are strong but tense, remember that you are not trying to develop more powerful muscles. Instead, you are trying to relax. These first exercises are more important for you than they are for anyone else.

GENERAL EXERCISES

No matter which K-W test or tests you failed, here are the six general exercises that you will use at the beginning and end of every exercise session. When you end your daily session, do your exercises in reverse order so that you conclude with the exercise with which you began.

To begin, strip down to your underclothes, take off your shoes and stockings, and lie on your back on a rug or pad on the floor. Get in a comfortable position. Put a pillow under your knees, a pillow under each arm, and another pillow or a rolled-up towel under the back of your neck. Now you are ready to start with the first exercise. Remember, you do each exercise two or three times and rest in between each.

EXERCISE 1.

Loosen up by wobbling your neck, your shoulders, arms, thighs, legs, and feet. Raise your arms slowly, then let them drop. Do the same with your hands, legs, and feet. Let your head drop to the left, then to the right. Take a deep breath—do not strain—exhale slowly.

Now try to feel heavy—let your head, shoulders, arms, and legs rest on the floor. Do not keep them up even slightly by tensing your muscles.

Breathe again, close your eyes, let your jaw sag, try to exhale as slowly as possible, humming or hissing.

Tighten your arm muscles, then let go. Do the same with your thigh muscles and neck, then let go. The important part is the letting go—not the tightening. The tightening is important only to make you feel the difference between tenseness and relaxation.

Breathe again, slowly lift your shoulders to your ears, let them go, shrug.

EXERCISE 2.

Get up, sit on chair, shrug your shoulders again.

EXERCISE 3.

Turn your head all the way to the left, then return it to normal front and center and relax. Turn all the way to the right as far as you can, return, and let go. If you have a stiff neck, do this while sitting as well as lying down.

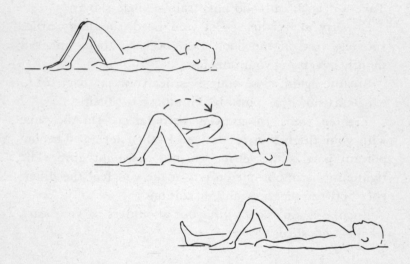

EXERCISE 4.

Lie flat on your back with all pillows removed, this time with your knees flexed. Slowly draw your right knee up as close as possible to your chest. Slowly straighten your leg, let it fall to the floor limp and relaxed. Pull it up again to the flexed starting position. Now do the same thing with the other leg. Alternate legs.

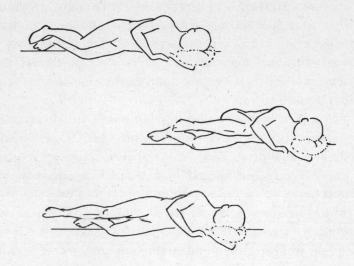

EXERCISE 5.

Lie on your left side, place a pillow under your head so it rests comfortably and your neck can relax. Keep both knees flexed and hips slightly flexed. Slide your right knee as close to your head as is comfortably possible, then slowly extend the leg until it is completely straight. Let the leg drop to the floor relaxed. Do the exercise two or three times on one side, then turn over to the other side and do the same with the other leg.

EXERCISE 6.

Turn over on your stomach. Fold your hands under your head and let your head rest on your hands comfortably. Then tighten your seat muscles. Hold for two seconds, then relax.

97

To repeat, these six exercises should be done, no matter what your K-W rating. After you have done all of these six general exercises in proper sequence you are ready to start additional exercises to correct your particular deficiencies. Add to your program one by one the exercises that pertain to you.

However, before you begin adding individual corrective exercises to the general six, read through the rest of this chapter. The prescribing of therapeutic exercises requires not only care but special knowledge. For instance, you must never do two sets of different exercises on your back, or on your stomach, consecutively. You must alternate each stomach exercise with a back exercise and vice versa. If you do not, you can stiffen and strain your muscles. It is as important to keep your muscles flexible as it is to keep them strong.

Furthermore, depending on which K-W test or tests you failed, each exercise program varies. Here, then, are descriptions and illustrations of the numbered exercises, from 7 through to 27, to be used to correct deficiencies revealed by the K-W tests. Read through them, study them, and see how they are done. Then, beginning later on page 112, pick the prescribed program for you. Then you will refer back to the exercises enumerated here.

CORRECTIVE EXERCISES

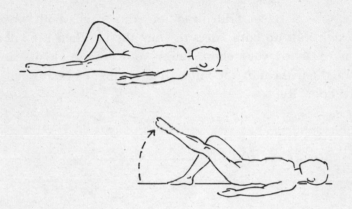

EXERCISE 7.

Rotated Leg Raise. Lie on your back with both knees flexed. Straighten one leg, turn the toes outward, and gradually lift the leg as illustrated. To make this exercise more effective, you will have to add weights when they are prescribed. You may use sandbags or light weight-lifting shoes. Start with two pounds, and do not add more than half a pound at a time every second or third day. As soon as you have to jerk or strain, the weight is excessive. Reduce it to the point where you can do it with ease and only slight effort. (This and the next exercise are principally used to strengthen weak hip flexors.)

EXERCISE 8.

Heel Slide. Lie on your back, both knees flexed. Pull up both knees to your chest. When the knees have reached your chest, lower your legs gradually and straighten them at the same time until they finally reach the floor. Relax.

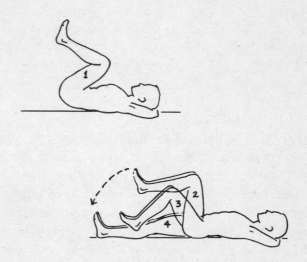

EXERCISE 9.

Abdominal Setting. Lie on your back, both knees flexed. Now tighten your stomach muscles. Try to tighten the seat muscles at the same time. If you do this correctly, the small of your back will be pressed against the floor. Do not do it by pressing with your legs. Let the tight muscles move your pelvis and bring your back against the floor. Do not push your back against the floor. You will not succeed at once. You may have to start by tightening your abdomen and later tightening your seat muscles separately before you can tighten them together. Once you succeed, hold muscles tight for two seconds, then let go.

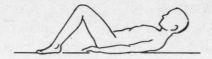

EXERCISE 10.

Head Up Supine. (This and the next two exercises are principally used to strengthen weak stomach, or abdominal, muscles.) Lie on floor, your knees flexed, hands loose by your side. Raise your head and shoulders off the floor, lower slowly and relax.

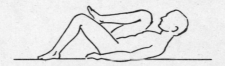

EXERCISE 11.

Knee Kiss. Lie on your back with knees flexed. Raise your head and your right knee at the same time and try to make them meet. Don't try too hard. You will probably not succeed. You will eventually. Return to your starting position and do the same with your head and left knee.

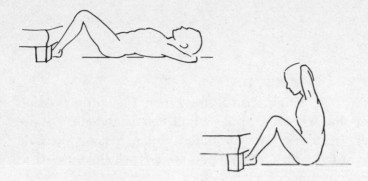

EXERCISE 12.

Sit-up, Knees Flexed. Lie on your back with your hands clasped behind your head, knees flexed. Tuck your feet under a chest of drawers, bed, or heavy chair. Be sure that the object is heavy enough so that it doesn't topple over. Sit up, then lower yourself slowly to lying position. You should sit up gradually, starting by raising your head, then your shoulders, and then your chest and lower end of the spine. Do not sit up by "hinging," that is, holding your trunk stiff and jerking your weight up. If you do not succeed in doing this exercise with your hands behind your neck, start by having them at your sides. Later, cross them over your stomach, and still later, when you are stronger, bring your crossed arms up to your chest and, finally, behind your neck and head. If you're unable to do this exercise at all, stick to earlier exercises until you have gained enough strength.

103

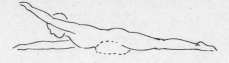

EXERCISE 13.

Single Arm Raise, Prone. Lie on the floor on your stomach with a pillow under your abdomen. Raise your right arm and shoulder, lower, relax. Alternate sides. (This and the next exercise are principally used to strengthen upper back muscles.)

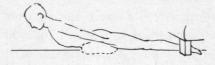

EXERCISE 14.

Back Up, Prone. Lie on your stomach with a large pillow under your waist. Anchor your feet under a heavy piece of furniture. Watch that the furniture doesn't topple on you. Keep your hands at your side. Raise your back. Raise your back until it is straight in line with your legs, but *do not* arch backward. (Arching back exercises, so-called hyper-extension exercises, have been prescribed frequently in the past and still are, but we have found that they can cause discomfort and pain in many cases. Backward arching is not a normal movement of the spine unless you're an acrobat. Do not do it.)

104

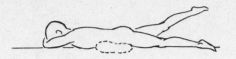

EXERCISE 15.

Single Leg Raise, Prone. Lie on your stomach with a large pillow under your waist. Raise one leg at a time, lower, rest. Alternate. (This and the next exercise are used principally to strengthen low-back and seat muscles. Note, however, that weakness of back muscles is very rare. If you cannot pass either of the back-muscle tests and fail other tests, too, you should definitely seek professional advice. Be sure to take the K-W tests with a sufficiently large pillow under your waist and be certain that your legs or upper back are respectively well anchored. If you don't anchor your legs and don't have a large enough pillow, you may not be able to pass, even though you are strong enough.)

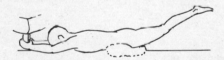

EXERCISE 16.

Double Leg Raise, Prone. Lie prone with a pillow under your hips. Anchor your hands by holding on to heavy furniture. Watch that furniture does not topple on you. Raise both legs at a time, lower, rest.

105

EXERCISE 17.

Prone Stretch. Lie on stomach, stretch left arm and right leg as far as you can along the floor, relax. Then do same with right arm and left leg. Then stretch with all four limbs at the same time, relax. (This and the remaining exercises are principally used to stretch muscles, from your shoulders to your hamstrings.)

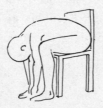

EXERCISE 18.

Bend Sitting. Sit on a chair, feet apart on the floor. Drop your neck, your shoulders, and your arms, then bend down between your knees, as far as you can. Return to upright position, straighten out, and relax.

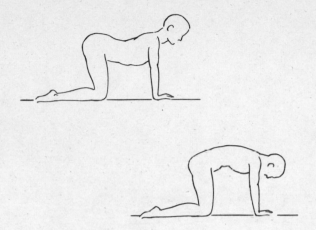

EXERCISE 19.

Cat Back. Assume a kneeling position, resting on your hands and knees. Arch your back like a cat, drop your head at the same time, then reverse positions by bringing up your head and sway-backing your spine.

EXERCISE 20.

Bend Sitting Rotation. Sit on chair as in "Bend Sitting" (Exercise 18). Bend down, dropping your head and shoulders. Bend down to the left, then gradually straighten up, rest. Do the same to the right.

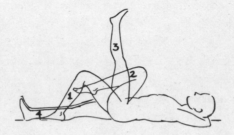

EXERCISE 21.

Hamstring Stretch. Lie on your back, both knees flexed, arms at sides. Bring one knee up to your face as close as possible, then raise your leg straight up in the air, then lower it slowly to the floor. As you do this you should feel a pull in your hamstrings. Return to starting position. Be sure that you relax before doing the same movement with the other knee.

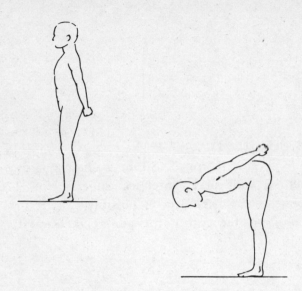

EXERCISE 22.

Hamstring Stretch Standing. Stand up, clasp your hands behind your back, keeping your back and neck straight. Gradually lower your trunk, bending from the hips, and go down as far as you can until you feel a stretching of your hamstring muscles.

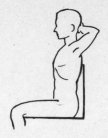

EXERCISE 23.

Pectoral Stretch. Sit in a chair, place your hands behind your neck, interlace fingers. Now bring your elbows as far back as you possibly can, return to starting position, then drop arms and relax. Repeat.

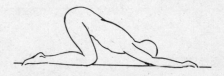

EXERCISE 24.

Kneeling Pectoral Stretch. Get on your knees and hands, then forearms, then gradually straighten out your back, sliding forward on your arms and keeping your back and head straight. This will stretch your pectoral muscles as you move away from your knees. Return to kneeling position, rest, repeat.

110

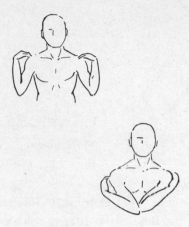

EXERCISE 25.

Upper Back Stretch. Sit on a chair with your hands on your shoulders. Try to cross your elbows by bringing your right arm as far left as possible and your left arm as far right as possible until you feel the stretch across your upper back. Return to starting position, drop hands, relax.

EXERCISE 26.

Shoulder Pull Prone. Lie on your stomach, pillow under hips. Pull your shoulder blades together and relax. This exercise can be helpful in combination with the "shrugging."

111

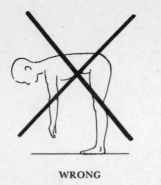

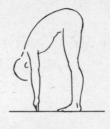

WRONG   RIGHT

EXERCISE 27.

Floor Touch. This exercise is identical with the K-W test (No. 6) for flexibility. It is the peak exercise given in all programs. To do it, first relax by inhaling and exhaling deeply. Drop your neck gradually and hang your trunk loosely from your hips. Drop your shoulders and then your back gradually. Let gravity help you. Do this two or three times. When you're completely relaxed, "hanging from the hips," try to touch the floor with your finger tips. Relax again, straighten up, then repeat.

Now that you have read through all the exercises, it is time for you to pick your prescribed program, a program prescribed to correct any deficiencies that have been revealed by the six K-W tests. Before you begin, however, remember that you should always take your time and that you should always start with general exercises 1 through 6 and conclude with them (and the rest of your program) in reverse order.

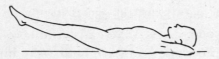

WEAK HIP FLEXORS

If you failed only K-W test 1 (shown here)—not being able to hold your heels ten inches above the floor for ten seconds—it is because you have weak hip flexors.

You will add the following exercises, one new one every two or three days, to the six general exercises: exercises 7 (without weight), 15, 7 (again, this time with weight), 19, 8, 18, and 27. Always do these exercises in this prescribed sequence, and when you have completed exercise 27, then return in reverse order to general exercise 1. Your full program, in order, will be exercises 1–6, 7, 15, 7, 19, 8, 18, 27, 18, 8, 19, 7, 15, 7, and 6–1.

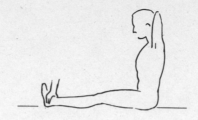

WEAK HIP FLEXORS AND ABDOMINALS

If you failed K-W test 2 (shown here), you are unable to sit up because you have both weak hip flexors and weak abdominals.

Weak abdominals, or stomach muscles, are tested in K-W test 3, and test 2 is included in the K-W series to gauge the relative weakness of hip flexors and abdominals at the same time. If you are weak in *both* hip flexors *and* abdominals, and still pass the other tests, you will add the following exercises, one new one every two or three days, to the six general exercises: exercises 9, 15, 10, 13, 11, 19, 12, 18, 22, and 27. When you are doing this full daily program, test yourself again. If you are able to pass K-W test 3 for weak abdominals, you probably will be able to pass K-W test 1 for weak hip flexors. But if you cannot pass K-W test 1, insert exercise 7 between exercises 18 and 22 and exercise 8 after exercise 27 in your program. You should always do all these exercises in this prescribed sequence and then return in reverse order to general exercise 1. Your full program, in order, will be exercises 1–6, 9, 15, 10, 13, 11, 19, 12, 18, (7), 22, 27, (8), 27, 22, (7), 18, 12, 19, 11, 13, 10, 15, 9, and 6–1.

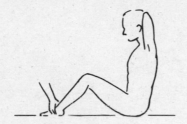

WEAK ABDOMINALS

If you failed only K-W test 3 (shown here), you are unable to sit up because you have weak abdominal, or stomach, muscles.

You will add the following exercises, one new one every two or three days, to the six general exercises: exercises 9, 15, 10, 13, 11, 19, 12, 18, 22, and 27. Always do these exercises in prescribed sequence, and when you have completed exercise 27, return in reverse order to general exercise 1. Your full program, in order, will be exercises 1–6, 9, 15, 10, 13, 11, 19, 12, 18, 22, 27, 22, 18, 12, 19, 11, 13, 10, 15, 9, and 6–1.

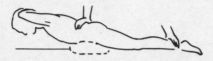

WEAK UPPER BACK

If you failed only K-W test 4 (shown here), you are unable to hold your trunk steady for ten seconds because you have weak upper-back muscles and should seek professional help, as previously indicated.

If your physician so advises, you will do the six general exercises and then the following exercises, one new one every two or three days: exercises 11, 13, 12, 17, 18, 14, 22, 24, and 27. Always do these exercises in prescribed sequence, and when you have completed exercise 27, return in reverse order to general exercise 1. Your full program, in order, will be exercises 1–6, 11, 13, 12, 17, 18, 14, 22, 24, 27, 24, 22, 14, 18, 17, 12, 13, 11, and 6–1.

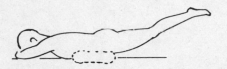

WEAK LOWER BACK

If you failed only K-W test 5 (shown here) and are unable to hold your legs up straight for ten seconds, you have weak lower-back muscles and should seek professional help as previously indicated.

If your physician so advises, you will do the six general exercises and then the following exercises, one new one every two or three days: exercises 11, 15, 12, 18, 16, 22, 19, and 27. Always do these exercises in prescribed sequence, and when you have completed exercise 27, return in reverse order to general exercise 1. Your full program, in order, will be exercises 1–6, 11, 15, 12, 18, 16, 22, 19, 27, 19, 22, 16, 18, 12, 15, 11, and 6–1.

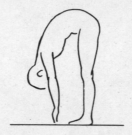

LACK OF FLEXIBILITY CAUSED BY TENSION AND STIFFNESS

If you failed only K-W test 6 (shown here)—inability to touch the floor with your finger tips—you are tense and lack flexibility.

You will add the following exercises, one new one every two or three days, to the six general exercises: exercises 12, 17, 18, 12 (again), 19, 11, 20, 21, 19, 22, 23, 24, and 27. Always do the exercises in this prescribed sequence, and when you have completed exercise 27, return in reverse order to general exercise 1. Your full program, in order, will be exercises 1–6, 12, 17, 18, 12, 19, 11, 20, 21, 19, 22, 23, 24, 27, 24, 23, 22, 19, 21, 20, 11, 19, 12, 18, 17, 12, and 6–1.

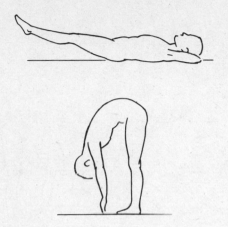

WEAK HIP FLEXORS AND LACK OF FLEXIBILITY

If you failed to pass both K-W tests 1 and 6 (shown here) but passed the other tests, you have both weak hip flexors and a lack of flexibility.

You will add the following exercises, one new one every two or three days, to the six general exercises: exercises 7 (without weight), 17, 18, 7 (again, this time with weight), 19, 20, 21, 22, 8, 23, 24, and 27. Always do these exercises in this prescribed sequence, and when you have completed exercise 27, return in reverse order to general exercise 1. Your full program, in order, will be exercises 1–6, 7, 17, 18, 7, 19, 20, 21, 22, 8, 23, 24, 27, 24, 23, 8, 22, 21, 20, 19, 7, 18, 17, 7, and 6–1.

119

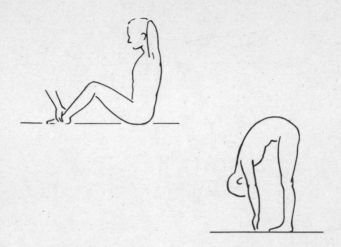

WEAK ABDOMINALS AND LACK OF FLEXIBILITY

If you have failed *both* K-W tests 3 and 6 (shown here) but passed the other tests, you have both weak abdominal muscles and a lack of flexibility.

You will add the following exercises, one new one every two or three days, to the six general exercises: exercises 9, 15, 10, 17, 11, 18, 12, 19, 20, 21, 22, and 27. Always do these exercises in prescribed sequence, and when you have completed exercise 27, return in reverse order to exercise 1. Your full program, in order, will be exercises 1–6, 9, 15, 10, 17, 11, 18, 12, 19, 20, 21, 22, 27, 22, 21, 20, 19, 12, 18, 11, 17, 10, 15, 9, and 6–1.

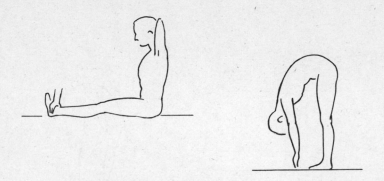

WEAK HIP FLEXORS AND ABDOMINALS AND LACK OF FLEXIBILITY

If you failed K-W tests 2 and 6 (shown here), you have not only weak hip flexors and weak abdominals, but you lack flexibility as well.

You will add the following exercises, one new one every two or three days, to the six general exercises: exercises 9, 15, 10, 13, 11, 19, 12, 18, 22, and 27. When you have reached this program, test yourself again. If you are able to pass K-W test 3 for weak abdominals, you probably will be able to pass K-W test 1 for weak hip flexors. If you cannot pass K-W test 1, insert exercise 7 between exercises 18 and 22 and exercise 8 after exercise 27. Always do these exercises in this prescribed sequence, and then return in reverse order to general exercise 1. Your full program, in order, will be exercises 1–6, 9, 15, 10, 13, 11, 19, 12, 18, (7), 22, (8), 27, (8), 22, (7), 18, 12, 19, 11, 13, 10, 15, 9, 6–1.

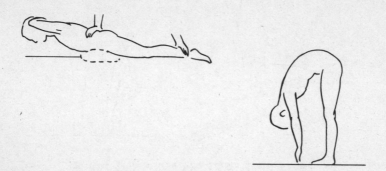

WEAK UPPER BACK AND LACK OF FLEXIBILITY

If you failed both K-W tests 4 and 6 (shown here), you have weak upper-back muscles and lack of flexibility. You should seek professional help as previously indicated.

If your physician so advises, you will do the six general exercises and then add the following exercises, one new one every two or three days: exercises 10, 13, 11, 19, 18, 14, 20, 21, 23, 24, 22, 25, 26, and 27. Always do these exercises in this prescribed sequence, and when you have completed exercise 27, return in reverse order to general exercise 1. Your full program, in order, will then be exercises 1–6, 10, 13, 11, 19, 18, 14, 20, 21, 23, 24, 22, 25, 26, 27, 26, 25, 22, 24, 23, 21, 20, 14, 18, 19, 11, 13, 10, and 6–1.

122

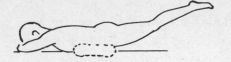

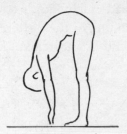

WEAK LOWER BACK AND LACK OF FLEXIBILITY

If you failed *both* K-W tests 5 and 6 (shown here), you have weak lower-back muscles and lack flexibility. You should seek professional help as previously indicated.

If your physician so advises, you will do the six general exercises and then add the following exercises, one new one every two or three days: exercises 10, 15, 11, 19, 18, 16, 20, 21, 22, and 27. Always do these exercises in the prescribed sequence, and then, after doing exercise 27, return in reverse order to exercise 1. Your full program, in order, will be exercises 1–6, 10, 15, 11, 19, 18, 16, 20, 21, 22, 27, 22, 21, 20, 16, 18, 19, 11, 15, 10, and 6–1.

SPECIAL ADDITIONAL EXERCISES

If you have been troubled by stiff neck or stiff shoulders, you may wish to add the following exercises to the end of your individual program (if they are not already included): exercises 23, 24, 25, and 26. In between each one of these exercises make sure that you shrug your shoulders and relax.

A NOTE OF CAUTION

If your K-W test failures do not fit any of the above combinations, you should again see your physician for a thorough review of your case. He will check on the possibility of pathology, trigger points, or fibrositis. If he excludes these as sources of trouble, he may compose a program for you, based on the exercises previously offered.

At long last, after consulting with your physician, you have embarked on your daily exercise program. Keep doing your prescribed exercises. Bear in mind, however, that although these exercises will bring you up to a level of "minimum muscular fitness," they will not make you fit for either heavy labor or demanding sports. These exercises do nothing whatever for your heart and circulation. They will help get you in condition, but you must add two new exercises, given below, before your activity has any effect on your heart and circulation. In addition to these two cardiovascular exercises, you should also engage in sports, a number of which are discussed in the next chapter.

Before you start the two exercises designed to increase the strength of your heart and circulation, make sure that your heart is in good shape and that your physician approves these exercises. A weak heart can be gradually retrained by exercise, but you should not try to decide this without medical advice.

CARDIOVASCULAR EXERCISE

1. Run in place. Raise your knees only slightly in the beginning and do the place running only for one or two minutes.

2. Stand with feet parallel, slightly apart; spread and stretch arms while inhaling; exhale, crossing arms in front of chest. After two or three times, go into a knee bend while exhaling and crossing arms, and return to standing position, inhaling with arms spread.

Pulse rate and breathing must increase in order to help the cardiovascular system.

3. Stand with your feet parallel, go into a knee bend (a half knee bend at first), then straighten up, and jump an inch off the floor.

Gradually increase the knee bends and jump higher. If your neighbors complain, or the people under you hear your jumping, you may do this exercise without jumping, but you have to increase the speed to make it effective. Do these exercises after you have gone through half of your regular daily exercise program, and then return and do those exercises in reverse.

After running or doing strenuous exercise you should feel hot and tired but not exhausted. The day after you should not have any pain or real discomfort in your muscles.

CHAPTER 7

Running, Yes; Golf, Maybe; Football, No

Now that you have started your exercise program, you must keep at it every day. When you are able to pass the K-W tests and are free from discomfort, you should also play sports or engage in some sort of vigorous physical activity to make sure that your muscles and heart get a good daily workout.

When you start playing sports, do so gradually. Do not rush yourself. Take it easy in the beginning, and build yourself up slowly. Above all, choose a sport or activity that will do you some definite good. Some sports are excellent, while others are harmful, even though they may seem pleasurable. When you take part in a sport, you should make certain that it is not only going to benefit you physically but emotionally as well. Some sports don't release tension. They add to it.

The basic sports, those that will put you in condition

and give you good physical and emotional workouts, are swimming, calisthenics, gymnastics, hiking, running and bicycling. Each of these, however, presents its own problems unless properly approached.

By far and away the best thing you can do is a lot of running. There is nothing that can match running—hard running—as a conditioner. If you start to run on a regular basis, you will get into excellent shape in no time. When your muscles no longer get stiff and tense after a workout, you may substitute running for your formal exercises.

It is not hard to find a place to run. Perhaps you live near a track, a school, or a Y.M.C.A. You can use a city park, a dirt road in the country, or even your own back yard. A lawn, a beach, or an open field will do. If the ground is gently rolling, it will add to the value of the workout. If you have not done any running previously, start easy and jog a distance until you feel winded or tired. You may warm up by walking awhile, then jog gently and walk again. After accustoming yourself to easy running, you may add brief faster periods so that in a month or two you can run a mile with little difficulty. In fact, any forty-year-old who has a good heart should be able to run two or three miles at an average of eight minutes per mile. I know much older people whose speed is faster than that and they do not get winded. Clock yourself so you can measure the improvement of your performance.

When you run, make certain that you warm up and cool off properly. Before and after you run, jog and walk. Work up a light sweat before you run; this is the sign that you are ready to go. When you have finished running, be

127

sure to limber your back muscles and legs and then stretch them. Several years ago I treated a number of college runners at our clinic. Four or five of them came in with torn hamstrings. When another one showed up, I phoned the coach, Mr. G. "Five or ten minutes is not enough time for a sprinter to warm up," I said. "Your boys should be hot and sweating before they run."

The coach didn't say much. He just listened, and when I was finished, he hung up with a brief "Thanks." I thought he was angry, and I was sure of it when he didn't send us any more of his boys.

Some time later I spoke at a college track coaches' luncheon in New York, and I talked about proper warm-ups. When the questioning started, who stood up but Mr. G.! I thought he was going to give me the devil. "Gentlemen," he said, "I just want you to know that a couple of years ago I sent a number of boys to the doctor's clinic. He told me that they weren't warming up properly. After that I never sent another boy to that clinic. I didn't have to—because I saw to it that the boys worked up a sweat before they ran."

Swimming is another sport that will get you in good shape provided you start slowly and increase your timing and distance by steps as you would in running. Swimming, of course, does nothing for you if you just take a dip and loaf in the sun. This is what many people do, and then they say they have had a workout.

Bicycling, too, is excellent for a vigorous workout. The same rules apply. Start gradually, don't overexert yourself, time yourself, and watch your distance if you're not used to it. You may be able to use a bicycle as transportation and so incorporate it into your daily activity. Be sure the handle bars and seat are properly adjusted so you don't crouch too much. When you pedal, you should straighten your knees completely, to stretch your hamstrings. Dr. Paul Dudley White, the heart specialist, is a great cycling enthusiast. He says he gets superb exercise from riding his bike, and at seventy-eight he should know.

Another basic sport is hiking. If you wish to do more than simply hiking over flat ground, look for hilly, rolling country or mountains. Hiking, especially with packs, can get you in shape if it is done regularly. If you hike at a brisk pace uphill or with a pack, it will do much for your cardiovascular system. Needless to say, any other activities involving hiking or running, such as hunting or chasing butterflies, are excellent too.

Gymnastics and calisthenics are excellent conditioners and should be taught in school. They do far more for overall development than do team sports, and they can keep you in good condition throughout life. They are true "carry-over sports." Unfortunately they have been dropped by many schools but there are still a few good teachers available. Without question, gymnastics and calisthenics should be revived and taught in every school.

Other sports and activities such as skiing, tennis, rowing, boxing, and chopping wood may help to keep you in condition, if you participate in them regularly. You have to be in shape to do these things. If you are in poor condition and participate, you run the risk of injury.

Skiing, of course, is a seasonal sport. In recent years it

129

has suffered from mechanization. Skiing is a good example of how we try to get the most pleasure from the least work. It has become mostly a chair-lift activity. No longer do you have to be able to hike up a slope before you can shoot down it. Unless you do warm-ups, you start your run cold (and often frozen after the trip in the lift), and so your first run down the mountain finds your body completely unprepared for any emergencies. If you like to ski, do some cross-country skiing, especially at the beginning of the season, and be sure to keep fit all year round.

Sad to say, skiing nowadays has become the sport of the non-athlete. A friend who leads a ski school in a resort near New York City told me that she had to refuse beginners who did not have enough strength to get up once they had fallen to the ground. I found it hard to believe her, but on my next visit to that resort I actually saw instructors reject several pupils who were completely unable to get up off the snow, even though the students were in the correct position to get up. This was true of a number of children as well.

Golf has lost much by mechanization. Golf carts have made walking unnecessary. One of the great fallacies about golf is the notion that it is a relaxing game. I am not overly sold on the game as a conditioner. Many patients say that they love the game because it "relaxes" them. It does not relax them, and it does not relax you. It *stimulates* you. Maybe golf does relax some people, for example, Arnold Palmer or Tony Lema on a day when they've shot a 66 in the opening round of the Masters or the U. S. Open. But you are not Palmer or Lema. A flubbed drive or a missed putt on one hole, and there goes your "relaxation." Do the same on the next hole, and you want to wrap your club around a tree. There can be no doubt that golf is an absorbing game, but it is absorbing because it is filled with mental tension from the first tee to the eighteenth green. I think the reason why golf is so popular with bankers, stockbrokers, and Presidents of the United States is because depressions, recessions, and even wars seem like small stuff after a bad round.

One of our patients, Fred W., was an ardent golfer. Or at least he was before he came to see us. Fred is in his late forties, has a beefy-red complexion, and is an account executive for an ad agency. Now, as you undoubtedly know, advertising is a frantic business. A new client comes in, and joy reigns. A client leaves, and half the office gets fired. It's up and down, from the heights to the depths, all the time. Advertising is a profession built on anxiety and tension.

Fred had been in "the agency game" for twenty years, ever since he graduated from one of the Ivy League schools. Advertising was his life and soul. He liked excitement, and he got it. He "relaxed" weekends playing golf; otherwise he got no exercise whatsoever, unless you count lifting a dry martini at lunch. If ever a man was designed for back pain, Fred was the man. He was tied up in knots with muscle tension, but he didn't think anything of it. Everyone he knew was in the same state. He thought tension was normal. In fact, he even thought he was in better shape than some of his colleagues because he didn't have ulcers.

One Friday, just as Fred was looking forward to a

weekend of golf, there was a meeting with a client. The client was a pest, and the agency had thought of resigning the account. But inasmuch as business was not then at its best, the agency kept the client, and poor Fred was the executive who had to deal with him. This Friday meeting was particularly exasperating. The client was complaining worse than ever. The meeting started at ten in the morning; it dragged on through lunch and didn't end until four that afternoon. Nothing was solved by the meeting. It had just been one long aggravation, and when it was over, Fred felt like punching not only the client but his boss as well for keeping the account.

Instead of doing either, Fred left the office with his anger bottled up inside him. He seethed all the way home on the train. The fact that the train was late did not help. When he got to his station, he didn't drive home but headed for a nearby driving range to let off steam. He bought a bucket of balls, lined them up on tees, and tried to smack each one as far as he could. Whenever Fred topped a drive, he would swing even more viciously at the next ball. He had hit about fifty balls when he felt a sudden stab in his lower back. He tried to hit another ball, but when he raised his driver, his left side seemed to become one massive, writhing knot of pain. He was frightened. He put down the driver and dragged himself to the car, his hand holding his back. He got home, and his wife helped him to bed. That is where he stayed until Monday morning when he hobbled into the clinic for help.

We looked at his back. His muscles were in severe spasm. Ethyl chloride and gentle limbering movements relieved some of his pain, and then we got his case history. We told him to go home and lie down and see us again on Wednesday. When he came back, we injected a trigger point in his low back with procaine. Fred had never heard of trigger points, so I told him about them. Then we discussed his case.

"I want you to do two things," I said. "When the pain eases, you must start on exercises to prevent it from coming back. This will make your back muscles flexible. As of now they are as stiff as a board. They are stiff with tension. You don't need any strengthening exercises. It's surprising, but you still have strength in your muscles. Your problem is tension. Now to help get rid of the tension, you should give up golf at least until I tell you it's all right to play."

"But I love golf," he protested. "It's my relaxation."

"It isn't," I said. "It's one of two sources of your tension. Your job is the other source. Would you rather give up your job?"

"No," Fred said.

"Then give up golf. When your back is in better shape, we'll see about golf. The chances are that you will be all right. Let's just see what happens."

Fred began his exercise program and kept faithfully at it. In two months' time he was coming along fine. He kept insisting that he wanted to start golfing again, and so after five months we let him go back to it. We were afraid that he would build up more tension from not being able to play. However, he now knows that he must exercise to keep tension down, and so he also swims three times a week at a health-club pool near his office.

Tennis is a good sport to keep you in condition. The important thing about tennis, or any other sport, is that you play regularly if you play at all. If you are overweight and forty and have just started one of the exercise programs described in the preceding chapter, do not rush out to play a hard game of singles or even doubles. Pace yourself. Be moderate. Then after you have gotten back into condition and have the knack of the game, start playing on a regular basis. By regular basis I mean once or twice a week at a minimum. Don't give up tennis for a month or two, and then suddenly get in a game on a Saturday morning and give it all you've got.

Fencing is another sport that will keep you in good condition, if done regularly. One drawback is that fencing is a "unilateral" activity; you use your body one-sidedly and thus you do not get an even workout. However, fencing does give you great tension release, and the activity is good for your cardiovascular system as well.

Much-maligned boxing can be a good carry-over sport, provided it is properly supervised and not done competitively. Boxing is often damned because professional boxing has been guilty of many ruthless practices. But that does not make boxing itself inherently bad. What I have in mind by boxing is a sparring session between partners of equal weight and skill. You can match opponents evenly, as you can in few other sports. You should make sure, of course, that the ring is sufficiently padded, that the gloves are of sufficient size to muffle the impact of the punches, and that head guards are worn.

The training required for boxing, such as punching the light and heavy bags, skipping rope, and running, is excellent for the system, and sparring in the ring, whereby you experience both tension ("Will he get me?") and release ("Ah, I got him!"), is most beneficial.

Many years ago, when I was still a young intern, a group of us used to exercise and box regularly with our friend and coach, Heinz Kowalski. At one time one of the boys was quite tense and more nervous than usual. He was getting ready to present his first paper to the local medical society. Obviously this was a great event, and he was tight and tense as can be. We all kidded him, but Kowalski took one look and said, "I'd like to spar a couple of rounds with you this afternoon before you start your great evening."

We had a good time watching Kowalski chase the young man around the ring, and pretty soon he seemed to have forgotten all about the impending ordeal. Only when he left the ring, warm, relaxed, and happy, did he notice that he had acquired a nice black shiner. The august members of the medical society might have wondered about this, but the young doctor's talk went off very well, with no hesitation or stumbling on his part.

Unfortunately our most popular sports are among the worst you can play. Football comes to mind at once, and I include touch football. Briefly put, football is legalized assault. A football game is not a contest between equals; a 150-pound halfback can be tackled by two or three 200-pound linemen. The chance for permanent injury is overwhelming. All too often a runner is clipped or hit from

135

behind. Piling on is a common abuse. I have yet to treat one ex-football player as a back patient who was not also bothered by a bad knee or shoulder injury.

In many ways touch football is worse than tackle. It is now becoming the weekend game for suburban middle-class males. More often than not, touch is played by men who are not in any sort of shape to start with, and as a result they are not prepared to withstand the sudden shocks and jars of the game. Touch football also builds tensions. Your neighbor gives you an extra hard block, and you retaliate. Before you know it, one of you is out of action with a broken wrist or arm and a bad temper. I know of one instance where a free-lance photographer didn't get any more assignments after he broke the shoulder of a magazine editor in the opposing backfield. If you wanted to see that editor get angry and tense, all you had to do was mention that photographer's name for the next six months. Whether touch or tackle, football is a game that requires great fitness but does not give you a chance to develop it.

Baseball cannot be viewed as a good game either for a sufficient physical workout. Most of the time the players, with the exception of the pitcher and catcher, simply stand around doing nothing at all. Then, all of a sudden, the center fielder, the third baseman, or the shortstop has to rush into action to field a ball, then wheel and throw to a base. Coming after a period of inactivity, this sudden burst of action can bring about injury. This applies equally to a base runner. One second he is standing idly near first; the

136

next second he's sprinting for third on a single, ready to slide to beat the throw.

Little League baseball does much more harm than good despite all the various excuses that have been made for it. Youngsters spend too much time playing baseball, time in which their bodies could be benefiting more profitably in far more vigorous pastimes. In addition, the intense competition can be harmful, particularly when the parents get emotionally involved and make the youngsters the pawns of their own egos. Go to a field and hear the parents carry on when a pinch hitter goes up in place of darling Junior or the umpire calls him out at home.

Intense baseball competition for youngsters is bad because it produces tensions, muscular and emotional, that cannot be relieved by the physical inactivity of the game. This holds true for the most talented youngster. He just cannot work off enough muscular steam in a ball game, and he may leave the field tense, no matter what the score or how many hits he got. Intense competition in any sport is bad for a growing child. It is especially bad for the youngster who, perhaps because of parental goading, has to push himself beyond his limits. When a child does this, he lays himself open to injury. He is playing under tension before the game even begins. This is true of some adults as well. Many of our patients are frustrated athletes. It is easy to spot them because they injure themselves repeatedly. We get skaters who cannot quite compete at the top level, but who push themselves nonetheless. We get the same skiers back time after time. They get hurt because they are not

137

very adept at skiing, yet they constantly try to push themselves beyond their abilities.

Of course, baseball is the national game, and it is natural for a youngster to want to play it. Let him play, but make sure that he gets regular and vigorous physical exercise beforehand. Exercise is the main course, and baseball, or any other sport for that matter, can serve as the dessert.

Volleyball, in many ways, is similar to baseball. It simply does not release the tension it builds up in a participant. Basketball is better, but it has come to be a game for the very tall, which means that it is a game for the very few. Not long ago I heard of a college basketball coach whose office door is six feet, four inches high. Outside is a sign saying, "If you can enter without stooping, don't."

There are any number of marginal sports that are popular but do little to keep you in good shape. They remain important for their recreational value. Bowling, horseshoe pitching, archery, sailing, and fishing, for instance, do not do you any physical harm, but they do not do you any physical good either. We know a patient who is absolutely smitten with fishing. He fishes almost every day. There is an excellent bass pond about a mile through the woods from his house, and he is there any chance he can get. He fishes the pond by wading. Sometimes his children—a girl, seven, and a boy, five—go with him. One day I asked him what he did in the way of sports. He told me all about his fishing. Did he tell me! I thought he would never stop as he described one leaping bass after another. Finally, when he calmed down, I said, "But that doesn't do you any good."

He spluttered and fumed. "Why, Doctor," he exclaimed, "fishing is the greatest relaxation a man can have!"

I had to agree that fishing was a fine mental relaxation. "Now I'll agree with you that the mind influences the muscles," I said, "but your muscles do not get a decent workout when you fish. In fact, from what you tell me, you spend too much time standing in one spot in your waders waiting for a bass to come by. Let me make two suggestions.

"The first is to move around a little more. Don't stand in one spot or hold one position with your body for more than ten or fifteen minutes. Even though you are relaxing, holding a certain body position is likely to make you tense even though you don't sense it. The other suggestion—instead of walking through the woods to the pond, run in."

"But I can't run in waders," he said.

"Carry them," I said. "Change when you get there. If you run in to fish, and run when you're finished, that will do you wonders. That and your daily exercise program should keep you free of tension."

He said he would try it. Now when he goes he often runs, and his children run along with him. It's a great game to him and a great game to them. And I know that when those youngsters grow up, they'll have not only an appreciation for nature and the outdoors but healthy muscles and strong hearts as well.

CHAPTER 8

Suggestions
for Daily Living

MANY PERSONS actually lead the life of a caged animal, often a tormented caged animal. They are plagued by irritations which they cannot fight or from which they cannot run. They fall victim to hypokinetic disease, to tension headaches, stiff neck, back pain, ulcers, heart trouble, and obesity.

You may be such a person. But once you start daily exercising and playing sports, you will have taken a giant step toward the prevention of hypokinetic disease. For once you will be doing for yourself what you usually expect others—the medical profession—to do for you: preventing disease. But this time it will be much harder than going to a doctor's office and just getting a vaccination, because the disease prevention is solely up to you. You are on your own with exercise. You have to do it yourself; you have to take the time for it.

Since you will be making a personal effort to avoid hypokinetic disease, you should also do all you can to stop irritations before they start.

You must always remember that irritations influence your mind and your mind then influences the muscles. Your mind and nerves work hard, and they work overtime. You live in a high-pressure society. Traffic lights, noise, commuter schedules, jangling telephones, missed appointments, a crying baby, a broken appliance—all these things and more subject your mind and then your muscles to repeated tension. You can work out this tension with your exercise program, but if you are smart, you will avoid much of the tension to begin with.

First of all, you must realize that you have become used to constant irritations, so used to them, in fact, that you don't notice them. You must recognize these irritations, however minor they may seem, and you must put a stop to them. For instance, if you are home and not forcibly subjected to irritations, you probably will turn on the radio. That radio noise in itself can be irritating. Then you may turn up the radio more, so as to drown out some vexatious street noise. That is doubly irritating. You probably keep the radio on even when you are talking to friends. Television will be going in one room and the radio in the next. You are so used to all this noise that you hardly concentrate on any of it. Yet this jumble of noise keeps diverting you, and you become used to drifting and being diverted. Your mind starts to feed on distractions and stimulants. You are eating the poison all the time without knowing it, and your mind and then your muscles become

141

needlessly alerted and tense. Sure, you are doing your exercises faithfully. Sure, you are running or swimming. Sure, you shed tension. But why let the tension get to you in the first place? You can stop it.

Take stock of your day. What external tensions bother you? Is it running to catch the train? Is it the children waking you up? Is it your teen-age daughter's record player blaring at odd hours? Make a list of these things, and rectify them. Don't run to catch the train. Get up earlier or catch a later train. Is it really that important that you catch that particular train? You must put things in perspective.

Take stock of situational tensions. Are you happy at work? Do you truly enjoy it? Do you get along with your boss or your employees? After you take stock you may find that some of these internal irritations are really not so annoying after all and that you can live with them peacefully. Look for the humor in a problem. Laughter breaks tension, and if you are able to laugh at yourself or smile to yourself at the foibles of your neighbors or fellow workers, you will do much to solve your problem. Then again, you may have to change what you are doing. You may have to let an employee go. You may want to ask for a transfer. You may have to change your job. The important thing is that you should be satisfied and happy in your life. If you are not, make a change. But if you cannot make a change, learn to accept. You are only hurting yourself by putting up with internal stress.

How is your home life? Here, too, changes can be made more easily than you may think, and they do not have to be drastic. You may wish to avoid visits from irritating friends or relatives or that annoying in-law. Your home is your castle, your place of rest. There is no reason why you should be disturbed if annoying visitors make you tense. You may have to give up living with your in-laws. You may have to stop forcing your son to become a lawyer when he really wants to be a teacher.

The most difficult task in dealing with sources of tension will be to solve inner emotional disturbances. All of us have problems, and for some of us they are serious. Exercise will ease tension, but exercise will not root out the cause of your tension. If you are willing to sit down with yourself and, instead of distracting yourself, concentrate on what irritates you, what upsets you, why a particular problem is hard to face, and what the alternatives are, you may be able to find the answer yourself. Then again, the source of your tension may be buried in some deep psychological disturbance, and you may need treatment for it.

That, of course, is up to you. Meanwhile you can avoid bad living habits that we have noted over the years. They can contribute to muscle tension, back pain, stiff neck, and nagging headaches. Some of these habits are so bad, in fact, that they may lock your muscles into a set position for most of the day, thereby greatly diminishing the effect of your daily exercise program.

Start the day leisurely. Eat a leisurely breakfast. Don't bolt your food. Don't let the children upset you. A bad temper in the morning can set your mood for the day. Don't read the paper and listen to the radio and keep an eye on the clock at the same time.

143

Dress comfortably. Much of the clothing and apparel for men and women almost seems deliberately designed to contribute to stress and tension. Shoes, especially women's shoes, can have a very bad effect. High heels often cause poor posture, shorten the calf muscles and hamstrings (which contribute to tension), and put too much weight on the forward part of the foot. A shoe with narrow toes makes the foot muscles rigid and tense. In turn your leg muscles will become tense and then so will your back muscles. Similarly, if your feet do not rest on a flat support, the foot muscles will tighten. Your foot should fit your shoe like a grasping hand. It should never be forced to become a hoof.

The heels of your shoes should fit well. They should not chafe up and down, nor should they "bite" into the ankle. Heels that are too loose or too tight will cause your ankles to sway, and the knees, hip joints, and neck can be affected. Shop around for your shoes. Sandals, by the way, are excellent. They give your toes free movement and gripping action.

Check your stockings. They are often too tight around the toes and thus interfere with the relaxation of your toes and feet. Your toes should not be restricted. You should be able to wiggle them freely.

Girdles are a hindrance to stomach muscles. If a woman is in good condition, she does not need to wear one. If she is not in good condition, she should try to build up her abdominal muscles so she can get along without support. A girdle is not only a concession to vanity; it is also a troublemaker. A tight girdle hinders natural trunk movements and turns the act of bending into a caricature.

144

Brassières with narrow shoulder straps can cause painful shoulder aches and pain in the upper back, partly by the direct pressure of the straps and partly by forcing the wearer into an artificially rigid position that just invites tension attacks.

Collars should always be loose. A collar that is too tight or too high can cause stiff neck or prompt a tension headache. Perhaps you will want to get your collars a half size larger. It will still look perfectly all right, and it will give your neck moving room.

Pajamas and nightgowns should be loose fitting. Don't let them restrict your sleeping movements.

Sleep on a firm mattress. Bed manufacturers are always shouting the praises of their wonderful mattresses and the marvels they will do for your back. But no matter what the ads claim, the best mattresses you can sleep on are made of horsehair, hog's hair, or felt, and they come without springs. A good mattress should be firm, should not give or sag, and above all, it should not hold the body in a groove that prevents you from turning freely during sleep. Inspect your mattress now. Does it measure up to these standards? If it does not, get rid of it. Whenever a patient is in the clinic, I always ask, "Do you sleep on a firm mattress?" The inevitable reply is, "Of course." I then ask the patient to sit on my couch, which is really a horsehair mattress. When they sit down and the couch doesn't yield, they usually jump up and exclaim how hard it is. "Well, that's how hard your mattress should be," I thereupon say.

If you have wide shoulders and sleep on your side, you

145

should have big enough pillows. Avoid foam-rubber pillows; they tend to keep your neck in a rigid position.

One low-back-pain patient, a salesman in his mid-thirties, used to sleep on a soft mattress. Once he started exercising, he changed to a hard mattress with a board underneath. Now, he says, he cannot sleep on a soft mattress at all. When he goes away on trips, he makes it a practice to ask the hotel to supply a bedboard. Bedboards are readily available, and hotels are glad to supply one if you request it. But sometimes this salesman still finds the bed too yielding. When that happens, he strips the sheets off the bed, puts them on the floor, draws a blanket over himself, and goes off to sleep. He did this recently when he was a house guest. His host thought it was rather strange, but the salesman says he had a wonderful rest on the floor.

Reading in an awkward position, be it peering closely at the print or holding the page at a distance, will bring on neck and back strain by forcing your muscles into an unnatural position. When you read, make certain that you are comfortable and that you have ample light.

Many persons get back or neck pain or stiffness from prolonged driving. If you are one of these persons, never drive more than one to two hours at a stretch. Pull over to the side of the road and walk around a bit. Relax. Shrug your shoulders frequently. You've been hunched over the wheel, and both you and your back muscles need a break. Look at the seat. It may be too small; it may also be too close or too far away from the foot pedals. Even if the seat is big enough and hard enough, you may still get back pain, because long-distance driving is conducive to tension.

Try to do your driving in easy stages. Don't rush. You'll get there.

Whether you are driving or staying still, sitting has its perils. Never sit in one position for more than an hour or two. If you have to do desk work, take an exercise break instead of a coffee break. Get up and move around. Keep your muscles limber. Don't let them get stiff. To take a quick breather, literally, inhale and exhale slowly three times. Shrug your shoulders a few times to loosen up tense neck and back muscles. Wobble your head from side to side. You may want to shift the position of your telephone. When it rings, your muscles go into alert. You get ready for fight or flight, and then you do neither. But you can react physically if you make it a practice to shrug when the phone rings. Instead of keeping the telephone always on one side of your desk, move it to the other side. Move it back and forth each day if possible. Give your muscles an even chance. Don't let the phone push you around.

Manual labor presents problems of its own. Usually there is not the mental tension that accompanies desk work, but in place of this are frequent and violent body movements. Carrying and lifting heavy loads are a frequent cause of back strain. Learn how to lift a heavy load correctly. You are lifting incorrectly if you bend over from the waist. You should bend from the knees instead if the load is heavy. If you are used to physical effort, you will be able to decide when a load is heavy for you and needs to be lifted carefully.

The constant handling of elevator doors, turning of handles, or repeated use of any instrument or machine may have telling effects on your muscles. Shoveling and using heavy hammers, especially when the blow strikes a hard surface, may cause all sorts of strain, especially in the upper extremities and in the shoulders. Vary your work routine. Break it up. Don't let it break you up. If you do not, detrimental effects are likely to occur, especially if you are not physically up to the job.

Whether day laborer, housewife, or executive, you should note what you are doing. Don't let yourself fall into a living pattern that invites tension. You can do a lot for yourself. Much tension is avoidable. By all means avoid it.

CHAPTER 9

The Diet Fad:
Eat but Exercise

THERE HAS BEEN MORE WRITTEN about eating and dieting than any single medical subject. No aspect of physical condition is of greater interest to the public than body weight. Obesity is discussed in innumerable books, pamphlets, magazines, newspapers, and on television. Overweight is a target for all sorts of commercial enterprises, whether they are special diets, reducing machines, or "gimmicks" to produce pinched waistlines.

Dieting has become a fad. You are told to start a crash diet, to start a gradual diet, to watch your calories, to eat fresh fruits and vegetables and cottage cheese, to avoid fried foods, to stay clear of starches, sweets, and fats. You are inundated with information and advice, much of it nonsensical.

There are exceptions to any rule, but there is one rule, solidly based on sound research, that applies to the great

149

majority of people who are not bothered, say, by glandular disorder or hereditary obesity. That rule is: *Eat as much as you want, but work off what you eat.* Obesity is most often caused by physical inactivity, not only by how much or what you eat. As a matter of fact, numerous studies have revealed that trim people often have a larger caloric intake than do people afflicted with obesity. As an additional rule I would suggest that you go easy on starches, avoid animal fats (use vegetable fats instead), and cut down on alcohol.

The main reason for your concern with overweight is because fat is aesthetically unpleasing. A trim figure is a must for a man or woman who wants to be presentable or attractive. Amazingly enough, to me, this desire for a trim figure is sometimes divorced from any wish for a physically fit and functional body. Such desire is based on personal vanity. You do not think of losing weight and keeping trim through exercise to improve your health and have a well-functioning body. Instead, you think of losing weight through dieting because you want to "look nice." This is fallacious thinking. You should remember, instead, that obesity increases mortality and the incidence of many diseases, including high blood pressure, arteriosclerosis, diabetes, and back pain.

Unfortunately the diet fad has become ingrained in American life. Even nutritional experts contribute to this fallacious idea by stressing diet alone rather than exercise. Back in 1958 the Food and Nutrition Board of the National Academy of Sciences issued recommended daily caloric intakes for the average American man and woman, who were named "reference man" and "reference woman."

Reference man, according to the Board's calculations, was twenty-five years old and weighed 154 pounds and was five feet nine inches tall. Reference woman was also twenty-five, weighed 128, and was five feet four inches tall. The Board advised that reference man consume 3200 calories a day and that reference woman eat 2300 a day to stay lean and "healthy." But in May 1964 the Board ordered reductions for both. Reference man was told to reduce his caloric intake from 3200 to only 2900 calories a day, and reference woman was told to cut her calories from 2300 to 2100.

Why? Because the Food and Nutrition Board decided that the average American man and woman—that's you—were not exerting themselves as much physically as they had in the past. Why didn't the Board advise them to exercise more? As a prominent medical journal remarked in reporting the Board's orders to reduce, "With the spread of power mowers, golf carts, and electric toothbrushes, the American way is fast becoming the Sedentary Way."

Instead of telling Americans to go on eating and exercise more, the Board told them to cut down on calories. This recommendation only adds to the problem. Underexercised people who diet often have the false and dangerous notion that they are in good condition. Furthermore, the Board's recommendations may be used as nutritional guides for hospitals, schools, and the Armed Forces, and many physicians will consult the Board's calorie counts for their patients, rather than advise increase of physical activity.

For twenty-five years exercise has been given no credit whatsoever by the diet faddists as having any role to play in weight control. In fact, exercise has been ridiculed and disparaged by the diet faddists, who have put forth a number of misconceptions to bolster their case. For instance, you often hear their argument that an increase in exercise leads to an increase of appetite and that exercise, therefore, is useless. This is false. Then again, you hear that you have to "split wood for seven hours" or "walk for thirty-six hours" to take off a pound of fat. This is true—but there is no rule saying that you have to split the wood in one session or do the walking at one clip. If you split wood for fifteen minutes a day or walk an hour a day as a regular practice, you burn up calories and lose fat. As a matter of fact, if you split wood for fifteen minutes a day every day of the year, you would lose twenty-six pounds of fat in a year. If you also played tennis regularly, you would burn up an additional fifteen to twenty pounds a year. Add the wood splitting and tennis together, and that's more than forty pounds a year. Of course it is ridiculous to expect you to do all this in one stretch, as the diet faddists imply, but when you spread the exercise over the days of the year, you will keep your weight under control at the same time you keep your muscles healthy. But the diet faddists do not tell you this.

Diet faddists will also tell you that if you do a great deal of physical exercise you will eat more. True enough, but you will not put on fat because you will burn off the calories. That is why soldiers in the field, day laborers, and many athletes can consume more than 6,000 calories a day and still be in the best of shape. As Dr. Norman Jolliffe says in his excellent book, *Reduce and Stay Reduced*, "muscular activity increases the caloric expenditure more than any other single factor." I am sure you have seen table after table showing how many calories there are in a steak, a martini, or an ice-cream sundae. On pages 154 and 155, for your constant reference, is something different, a table of energy expenditure compiled by Dr. Jean Mayer of the Harvard University School of Public Health. Dr. Mayer is one of the country's foremost nutritionists, and the table will show you how many calories you use up in an hour in various activities. Check to see how you are doing and what you can do to burn off more.

There have been any number of interesting experiments on the effect of exercise on eating. A few years ago Harvard students were asked to double their daily food intake, from 3,000 to 6,000 calories. With all their classroom work the students were hard pressed to find the time to exercise, but they did exercise and they managed to "lose" the extra 3,000 calories per day.

Dr. Mayer conducted an extensive study on carefully paired groups of obese and trim suburban high-school girls. Particular attention was paid to a systematic comparison of caloric intake and physical activity in both groups. He found a marked difference between the fat girls and the trim girls. The trim girls were physically active; the fat girls were less than half as active. Even so, the trim girls generally ate more than did the fat girls, leading Dr. Mayer to the logical conclusion that being inactive contributed more to obesity than overeating. Ironically Dr. Mayer discovered that the fat girls were often excused from sports upon recommendation of physicians.

Similar findings have been made by other researchers.

CALORIE REQUIREMENTS FOR VARIOUS ACTIVITIES*

Activities	Calories Per Hour
DOMESTIC OCCUPATIONS	
Sewing	10–30
Writing	20
Sitting at rest	15
Standing relaxed	20
Dressing and undressing	30–40
Ironing (with 5-lb. iron)	60
Dishwashing	60
Sweeping or dusting	80–130
Polishing	150–200
INDUSTRIAL OCCUPATIONS	
Tailoring	50–100
Shoemaking	80–100
Bookbinding	75–100
Locksmithing	150–200
Housepainting	150–200
Carpentering	150–200
Joinering	200
Cartwrighting	200
Smithing (light work)	250–300
Smithing (heavy work)	300–400
Riveting	300
Coal mining (avg. for shift)	200–400
Stone masoning	300–400
Sawing wood	400–600
PHYSICAL EXERCISE	
Walking	
2 mph	200
3 mph	270
4 mph	350

Activities	Calories Per Hour
Running	800–1000
Cycling	
5 mph	250
10 mph	450
14 mph	700
Horseback riding	
Walking	150
Trotting	500
Galloping	600
Dancing	200–400
Gymnastics	200–500
Golfing	300
Playing tennis	400–500
Playing soccer	550
Canoeing	
2.5 mph	180
4.0 mph	420
Sculling	
50 strokes per minute	420
97 strokes per minute	670
Rowing (peak effort)	1200
Swimming	
Breast and back stroke	300–650
Crawl	700–900
Playing squash	600–700
Climbing	700–900
Skiing	600–700
Skating (fast)	300–700
Wrestling	900–1000

Figures obtained for 150-lb. subject.

* Modified from J. B. Orr and I. Leitch, "The Determination of the Caloric Requirements in Man," *Nutrition Abstr. & Rev.*, 7:509, 1938; and R. Passmore and J. V. G. A. Durnin, "Human Energy Expenditure," *Physiol. Rev.*, 35:801, 1955, by Dr. Jean Mayer.

Dr. J. A. Greene studied more than two hundred overweight adult patients and found that the beginning of their weight problems was directly traceable to a sudden decrease in physical activity. Dr. Hilda Bruch studied 160 fat children, and inactivity was characteristic of the great majority; 88 per cent of the girls and 76 per cent of the boys were inactive. Danish researchers came up with much the same results in studies they made. I could cite one study after another, all by responsible scientists; they all show that it is not how much you eat but how much you exercise.

A diet may, of course, be essential in combination with exercise. Here is a sample case. One morning a salesman named Donald D. came into the clinic. I should say he waddled in. He was five foot nine, and he weighed 242 pounds. He was thirty-seven years old. His weight, for his build, should have been 170 pounds. Mr. D. was suffering from chronic back pain. His muscles had become too weak to support his weight. Like most fat people, be they unhappy children, depressed housewives, or anxious executives, he tried to make up for his frustrations by eating and eating and eating. Since he did no exercise whatsoever, he became a balloon.

There was no point in seeing if Mr. D. could touch the floor. Even if he did not have tight back muscles and hamstrings, he never could have gotten past his bulging stomach. We started him on an exercise program, and to hasten recovery, he was also put on a strict diet. As it was, it took a solid year to get Mr. D. down to 170 pounds and his muscles in good shape. If he had not been put on a diet, he could have waited forever for his weight to reach normal.

Once Mr. D. got his weight down, he took up swimming and tennis. Now he keeps up his physical activities, having learned that they are a need, not a luxury.

I would like to conclude by citing Dr. Mayer again. What he says is of the greatest significance for you. He writes:

"The author is convinced that inactivity is the most important factor explaining the frequency of 'creeping' overweight in modern Western societies. Natural selection, operating for hundreds of thousands of years, made men physically active, resourceful creatures, well prepared to be hunters, fishermen, or agriculturalists. The regulation of food intake was never designed to adapt to the highly mechanized sedentary conditions of modern life, any more than animals were made to be caged. Adaptation to these conditions without development of obesity means that either the individual will have to step up his activity or that he will be mildly or acutely hungry all his life. The first alternative is difficult, especially as present conditions in the United States, especially in cities, offer little inducement to walking and are often poorly organized as regards facilities for adult exercise. Even among the young, highly competitive sports for the few are emphasized at the expense of individual sports which all could learn and continue to enjoy after the high-school and college years are over. But if the first alternative, stepping up activity, is difficult, it is well to remember that the second alternative, i.e., lifetime hunger, is so much more difficult that to rely on it for weight-control programs can only continue to lead to the fiascos of the past.

"Strenuous exercise on an irregular basis, in untrained individuals already obese, is obviously not what is advocated. But a reorganization of one's life to include regular exercise adapted to one's physical potentialities is a justified return to the wisdom of the ages."

CHAPTER 10

What Can You Do
for Your Children?

ANY DISEASE produced by lack of exercise is a deficiency disease. As such—like a vitamin deficiency—it hits hardest at the young.

Few mothers will forget to feed their children enough vitamins—but how many will see to it that they have enough exercise? Few parents will miss having their children vaccinated against smallpox, diphtheria, polio, and other contagious diseases, but how many even think of preventing hypokinetic disease? Still, lack of sufficient exercise and good exercise habits instilled in childhood is the main cause of tension pain, back pain, overweight, and heart disease in later life. Geriatrics starts in the cradle. It is up to the parent, then the school and the community, to do something about this. Yet they rarely do. The importance of this is not understood. Moreover, too many physicians and educators regard exercise and vigorous physical

159

activity as a "frill" rather than a basic human need. Parents believe them and, if they are not active themselves, go along with this dangerous thinking. If you are a parent, you must see to it that your children engage in vigorous physical activity not only at home but also at school, whether it be kindergarten or college.

Children are the first to suffer in our sedentary society. When you and I were youngsters, we did not have automobiles, television, and appliances galore. If you are flabby or tense, you can rectify this because you at least built the semblance of a body in your childhood. But your children are different. Your children do not lead the comparatively vigorous life that you led. Their muscles rarely get a workout, and their muscles do not develop properly. Instead of walking, today's youngsters ride. Notice the next time your boy or girl wants to go somewhere. Even if it is just down the street, they'll ask you to give them a lift. And the bad part of this situation is that you don't think anything of it.

Think of the hours upon hours children spend staring at television. Recent studies reveal that high school teen-agers spend up to thirty hours a week watching television and only two hours exercising. Even if every program were excellent—and I am sure you will agree that often the opposite is the case—the time spent is harmful. Television and radio programs build up tension in a child at the same time that they keep him from having a physical outlet. You should no more let your child saturate himself with television or radio or similar sedentary distractions than you should expose him to a contagious disease without inoculation. This may sound harsh, but it is the truth. The muscular condition of the majority of American youngsters is appalling.

You can find out if your children have minimum strength and flexibility by giving them the K-W tests. If they do not pass all of them, this means they are not active enough, that they get more irritations than they can work off, that they watch more than they play, and that they are establishing a damaging lifelong pattern. You ought to change this. See to it that they run, that they swim, that they walk, and play games requiring lots of action. See to it that your child learns the feeling of physical effort and physical accomplishment. This—in our growing, hectic, urban society—can best be accomplished not only at home but in disciplined exercise classes. There the first roots of discipline—not regimentation—can grow; there the teacher can pay special attention to individual needs. If you have no classes available, band together with other families and hire a good exercise or ballet instructor for your group of children. Dance classes for even three-year-olds are excellent.

Children like to imitate their elders, and if you lead a physically active life, you will find that your children will want to do what you do. In this way physical activity will come naturally and easily for a child. It will be like breathing. When you go out to swim, hike, run, skate, or ski, let your child come along.

You can start with the baby. Instead of imprisoning him in a confining playpen, stick him out on the lawn and let him move around. Let him try out his muscles; let him develop them at a natural pace. If your baby does not walk

161

as soon as the others in a neighborhood, don't worry. The crawling about does him a great deal of good; it gives him the opportunity to develop strong trunk muscles. As he grows older, let him climb trees and fences if he wants to. Too many parents—all too often the same parents who *push* their children into a sport—are afraid their children will hurt themselves. If a boy or girl breaks an arm, true, it may be in a cast for a while. That is not the worst catastrophe. The real danger is in not letting the child learn about physical dangers. In point of fact, the child that does not have the chance to learn about danger is often the child who is likely to suffer severe injury.

Do not be overanxious. Of course, at the same time do not be reckless. There is a dividing line between the two. Let me give you an example. I know a couple, parents of a young daughter, who do a lot of skiing. When the girl was only three, she said she wanted to ski, too. Her parents neither pushed nor discouraged her. Instead, they simply gave her a pair of skis to use around the back yard. Soon the little girl asked to accompany them skiing. Finally one weekend they gave in. They took her up the beginner's slope, then they let her loose. She schussed down, with her parents at her side to make sure that she did not hit a tree or a rock. The little girl couldn't get enough, but her parents took her off the slope before she had a chance to get bored or tired. They did this for a number of weekends, always making her walk up the slope, and continued this routine the following winter. At the age of five she was ready for ski school. Today this little girl is developing into an excellent skier. More important, she has started to use her body. She learned to ski because her parents did, because she wanted to, and because she had parents who knew how to handle the problem. There is all the difference in the world between setting an example for children and pushing them into an activity for which they have no desire.

Children forced into a sport often rebel, especially if they are below par physically. Recently I saw a twelve-year-old boy, whose parents brought him in to the clinic because they were alarmed about his "poor posture." There was nothing radically wrong with this boy—he had no organic diseases—but he hunched his shoulders and had what can only be described as a hangdog look, common in children and adults who are depressed or frustrated. When I tested the boy, I found that he had weak abdominal muscles and that his lower-back muscles and hamstrings were stiff and rigid. All in all, he was extremely tense. You could see the prospective back pain developing right then and there. Obviously corrective measures were necessary.

I talked to both the boy and his parents, and the parents soon made it evident that while they were both active and athletic, the boy was listless. When he first went to school, he tried to make a class team but failed, even though he worked hard. This pattern kept up for the first few years in school, and he always competed unsuccessfully. By the fourth grade he hated anything connected with sports, and he used every possible excuse to avoid the merest hint of exercise. Of course, the more he balked the more his parents pushed him. He developed "poor posture" as a defense, and then his parents grew concerned.

I could tell that the boy was embarrassed at being seen by a doctor. It was bad enough that he was "no good" at sports, but now he had to see a doctor because something was "wrong" with him. To spare the boy further embarrassment that could only worsen the problem, I told the parents that I was going to send him to an exercise teacher. In the beginning he would do the exercises only with the teacher. Then, after he had learned the exercises thoroughly, he would do them in a compatible group. There would be no competition whatsoever, and I told the parents not to push him. As a result of working with an exercise teacher, the boy made excellent progress. His back and posture improved considerably, and his attitude changed. Now he plays sports, and although he is far from the best athlete in the world, he is a healthy youngster with a positive attitude toward vigorous exercise.

It really is easy to keep your children physically active at home; it becomes difficult when they start school. As long as they are infants and pre-schoolers, all you have to do is avoid suppressing their natural urge to move. But then comes school, and many school systems have very poor physical education programs. From an athletic point of view we have the most undemocratic schools in the world. A school can have as many as three to four thousand students, but the only ones who receive systematic muscular training are those who have won a place on one of the varsity athletic teams. This is contrary to common sense, which tells you that the children who are the least exercised are the ones who need it the most.

Instead of lavishing attention on the gifted athletes, schools should institute broad, non-competitive exercise programs that benefit all the students. This does not mean that competitive sports should be neglected. Sports have their place, but that place comes after the physical needs of the over-all student body have been met. That should be the aim of physical education.

I consider this so important that I think it is worth repeating: Instead of picking the most physically gifted and welding them into winning teams for the glory of the school (and the coaches), the emphasis should be on all the students. Then, if after years of systematic training, a few emerge with special talents, they should be encouraged to make their mark as competitive athletes.

Systematic physical training should start in kindergarten and continue through elementary school, high school, and college. Sports programs should be the icing on the cake, and they should be selective. Physical education for all should consist of one hour a day of formal training, including calisthenics, gymnastics, running, and swimming. Parents should make sure that this period is really one full hour. All too often school administrators skimp on this; it is often the first time period they cut. Studies by Dr. Josephine L. Rathbone of Columbia University indicate that only twenty minutes of each school hour assigned to physical education are actually utilized. Make sure this is not happening in your school.

Exercise programs should be compulsory. I know exercise is all too often taught without imagination. If taught properly and with a purpose, and if the participants are kept busy all the time, it is attractive to youngsters. They love to play leapfrog, tumble, chin themselves, and climb ropes. Exercise has to start early in life; if a child has become sedentary and sluggish before the age of six, it will be hard for a teacher to rouse his interest. And it is exactly this type of child that needs special attention and care.

The exercise class can be used to teach discipline, an area which is neglected if not ignored in schools because it is usually confused with regimentation. From easily understood and amusing exercises like bunny hops and cat crawls children can be gradually brought to accomplish more difficult movements. In short order they will be able to carry out "difficult" exercises. As soon as possible exercises should challenge their strength, their endurance, and their coordination. The more challenging they are, the more interesting they will be.

A young child should learn to improve his abilities without actually competing with other children. He should measure his own improvement, not compare his performance with that of another. Children grow at different rates, and competition should come in later childhood, say after twelve, and then competition should be encouraged only when it buds spontaneously. To force a young child to compete when the contest is hopeless and the child knows that he is destined to be a loser will do the child no good. There is nothing more disheartening to a youngster, and he falls into the lifelong habit of always doubting himself.

Above all, the teacher should set the example. He or she

should be fit, should come to class in gym clothes, and should work personally with the children. He should not only be able to do what they do, but he should be able to do any exercise better than they can. When we administered the Kraus-Weber tests to children in Zurich, we talked to many local physical educators. I was impressed by their athletic appearance, and I was especially impressed by the oldest of them, a sixty-five-year-old man who was the chief of the local group. When I asked him whether he still worked actively with the children, he replied, "Yes, of course. I have to, because the moment I cannot chin myself better than the next youngster, and as soon as I cannot run and jump with them, I cannot function as a practical teacher, and I do not want to retire to theory at this stage."

By contrast, I remember an occasion when a friend, an excellent teacher in physical education, had to attend a dinner at a well-known university. I went with him as a guest. The dining room was on the second floor of the physical education building, and the only elevator was very small. There was a great crowd of physical educators waiting on the first floor to crowd into the jammed elevator. Only a few of them decided to walk the flight of stairs to the dining room. As we walked up the stairs my friend said, "I am afraid that with so few using the stairs, physical education is still missing the first goal."

In the dining room I noticed that most of the physical educators were either overweight or stooped. There were a few with trim, athletic figures, but unfortunately very few. On the whole, the gathering did not look any different from any clambake of underexercised office workers. Why was this? Because in physical education there is more interest in methodology and theory than in actual doing. Since actual doing, actual moving, and actual exercising are only a small part of the curricula of the average physical education school, it is small wonder that the graduates do not look different from any other students who have spent four years sitting in a library. The basic need in physical education is a change of attitude. The basic need here is for acceptance of the physical as an important and essential base for the intellectual and not as a secondary afterthought. Because of efforts by dedicated physical educators such as Frederic R. Rogers, Harrison Clark and others, there are some schools with good programs. Springfield College and Boston College for Physical Education are moving in the right direction; they stress the actual physical participation of the students.

Recently I was a speaker at the Physical Education Department at San Diego State College in California. When the morning program was over, I was asked to join the routine noon workout. The whole faculty, including the department head, Dr. Fred Kash, changed to gym clothes and joined the students for very active exercise programs. After a half hour of this everyone ran two miles on the campus lawn. The participants included graduates who had come back to see what was new, and I feel that they learned a lot. The afternoon session closed with a similar procedure, only this time swimming was added. The Physical Education Department works with schools and children in the growing San Diego area, and it has performed a truly remarkable job in a short time.

Unfortunately, in contrast to San Diego's excellent programs, there are other schools where physical education is taken up by students because it is the "easiest" course and a degree gives a graduate an entree into the school systems as an "administrator." Such an administrator may have very little love for the actual physical improvement of his children.

Besides exercises, the daily school program should include healthy doses of calorie-burning activities, such as running, jumping, and swimming. Youngsters should get a well-rounded and vigorous workout every day at school. Intramural sports programs should not start until the fifth or sixth grade, and when they do start, the intramurals should be optional and held after school hours, as should be the case with varsity sports. In short, no sports activity should be allowed to replace or supplant the basic daily exercise program.

To those who claim that strong physical education programs and strong discipline smack of the totalitarian state, I would like to point out that Switzerland, the oldest existing democracy in the world, has a model program. The government sets the requirements to insure a basic national standard. Youngsters are graded and must pass annual tests, and the results of the tests are recorded in a booklet for each student. Upon graduating from high school a boy receives his booklet and then, in turn, presents it to the authorities in charge of military training. If his marks do not meet the minimum physical requirements, he receives special training before induction. Furthermore, a boy is not eligible for officer's candidate school unless his marks

169

show that he can meet high standards. Girls are given similar physical-fitness tests in school, and although they do not have to serve in the army, the example set by the boys makes them adhere to the standards.

It is interesting to note that the Swiss have national standards. We do not have national standards for physical fitness or any other scholastic requirements. In his book *Swiss Education and Ours,* Admiral Hyman Rickover points out that this lack of minimum national standards is a great drawback. National or federal standards could be set without interfering with local school boards.

The minimum requirements set by Swiss schools and the government are not nearly as minimal as the word makes them sound. Besides their regular school training, children give over one afternoon a week, usually a Saturday afternoon, to an outing with the teacher. The whole class swims, hikes, and camps together. In addition, children are required to walk to school. Only those who live more than two miles from school are allowed to use streetcars or even bicycles. The Swiss authorities are very much aware of the influence of increasing mechanization, and they take every opportunity to offset it where it may harm or hinder the physical development of the young.

A specific instance of the careful Swiss attitude comes to mind. When we set out in 1952 to administer our tests to American and European school children, we had, of course, to secure permission from school authorities concerned. The receptions we got varied in different cities. When we asked for permission to test children in one very large

American city, we were given evasive answers. A school official finally came out with the real reason for refusing us permission. "Why, we can't possibly let you do this," he said. "Suppose you find out our children are not as fit as they should be. Then what are we going to do?"

By comparison, in Zurich we got cooperation almost immediately. After we explained what we wanted to do, the medical officer in charge of the school system said he would be delighted to give us permission. He called in his aides and told them to give us all possible assistance. He saw to it that all the schools were notified. Then he gave us a breakdown of the school system, so that we could test a cross section of Zurich's children, from rich to poor. After he had done all this for us, he said that he only had one request, and that was that we were to inform him fully of our findings so that he could apply any corrective measures needed.

Without question, we need to revamp physical education in our schools. Physical education has never gotten the overhaul that the academic curriculum got when Sputnik went up. Indeed, when we all became aware that an intensifying drive for quality education was necessary, this was frequently done at the expense of physical training. Not long ago the California legislature considered abolishing physical education as a requirement. In an attempt to prevent this, proponents of physical education stressed the point that physical education was needed to prevent an increase in hypokinetic disease. Much of the material that my associates and I had gathered, including our K-W test

171

results, was offered as one of the arguments to prevent the change of law. The bill failed.

A revolution in physical education is crucially needed if youngsters are to be safeguarded from hypokinetic disease.

CHAPTER 11

What Can Be Done
for Our Country

TREATMENT OF A BACK-PAIN and tension patient often lasts for months and sometimes a year or more. It is always pleasing when the patient recovers and returns to a full and active life, but the question always occurs to us, was all this effort, all this time, and all this suffering necessary? Could not all this have been prevented? The answer, for the vast majority of cases, is yes. Disease produced by lack of exercise is preventable. And yet we have no sooner finished with one patient than there are two more waiting for treatment. The flood seems never-ending.

Why does it continue? Because programs for adults are practically nonexistent. We can talk about what parents should do and what the schools should do, but so far very few have talked about what can be done for adults. Happily I believe that something, something positive, can be done, not merely to cure underexercise disease, but to prevent its

173

occurrence in the first place. This we must do if we are to handle the problem intelligently.

The United States leads the world in the prevention of contagious disease. It lags behind other advanced countries in the prevention of hypokinetic disease. Our medical scientists, philanthropic foundations, and social scientists seem unaware of the fact that for years a number of European countries, on both sides of the Iron Curtain, have been carrying on programs to prevent hypokinetic disease. These programs are backed by private industry, labor unions, insurance companies, and governments. In country after country reconditioning centers have been established to offset the dangers brought about by mechanization in living.

Surprisingly, one of the countries most deeply committed to the prevention of hypokinetic disease is the Soviet Union. The results have been impressive, so much so that the former Soviet Minister of Health, Madame Kovrigina, has boasted that for every death caused by heart disease in the U.S.S.R. there have been more than two such deaths in the United States. I cannot evaluate the validity of this Soviet claim, but I do know for a fact that in the Soviet there are more than 2,500 reconditioning centers treating at least five million patients a year. These patients are put through reconditioning programs as part of the government's program of "physical culture." In addition, there are a great many "night sanitoria" attached to larger industrial plants, where overtired and tense workers are assigned for three weeks during off hours. When you consider

174

the fact that the Soviet Union, which does not have anywhere near the prosperous (and underexercised) society
that we have, has recognized and is coping with the problem, you may well wonder why no action has been taken
in this country.

The Soviet satellites of Czechoslovakia and East Germany also maintain numerous reconditioning centers. A
few years ago East Germany instituted a seven-year plan
for health preservation, with the goal of eventually reconditioning one million sedentary persons a year. By contrast,
in the United States, prevention of disease through exercise has been practiced at an academic level at best. We
need comprehensive reconditioning centers to combat hypokinetic disease at its onset. They would form an important part of President Johnson's program to combat heart
disease and stroke.

West German centers might serve as logical models for
institutions in this country. Socio-economic conditions and
the incidence of hypokinetic disease are similar to our own,
and there are eleven years' worth of detailed reports on
organization, methods, and experience that we can draw
upon for study.

Dr. Peter Beckmann has been the pioneer for the prevention of hypokinetic disease in West Germany. In 1953
he set up a reconditioning center in Ohlstadt, Upper
Bavaria, for two hundred sedentary persons. The Ohlstadt
center was so successful that others followed; there are
fifteen reconditioning centers operating in West Germany
at this writing. They are supported by insurance companies

and industrial enterprises, such as Opel Automobile, Mannesmann Steelworks, Siemens Halske Electric Works, and various Ruhr mining companies.

Treatment at the centers is free, and the patients receive up to 80 per cent of their regular salaries, depending upon family circumstances. The time spent in a reconditioning course does not count against vacation time. This might seem prohibitively expensive, but the centers more than pay for themselves, as work absenteeism through physical disability has been cut in half.

Admission to a center is based upon the recommendation of an applicant's insurance physician and a statement from the applicant's supervisor, indicating that his work performance has regressed. Medical indications are liberal; the patient does not have to be in acute distress. He may be admitted on the basis of minor problems, including subjective complaints concerning the cardiovascular and muscle systems, the digestive tract, insomnia, general fatigue, premature aging, and so on. Each patient has to present a complete pre-admission certificate and, in turn, when he leaves he receives a report for his regular physician. If rejected for treatment, an insured worker has the right of appeal under West German law.

Although the centers put the primary emphasis on systematic and intensive exercise programs, they give careful attention to psychological and emotional factors. The centers are intended to help tense, irritated, emotionally overstrained and fatigued patients from factories, shops, offices, and mines "get away from it all." The centers are situated in scenic areas, near mountains, forests, or sandy beaches. They offer plain but pleasant living quarters and are equipped with gyms, indoor and outdoor swimming pools, social halls, and sauna baths. In short, the atmosphere is congenial and mentally relaxing, and everyone has the chance to enjoy the beauty and invigorating influence of nature. To a good many patients this is an entirely new experience.

At Ohlstadt the daily program consists of systematic calisthenics and breathing exercises, running, swimming, bathing, and ball games during the morning and an hour or two of relaxation after lunch. More games, hiking through the countryside, and climbing occupy the afternoon. The evening hours are given over to health discussions, lectures, lessons in crafts and hobbies, and cultural presentations. Radio and television are barred as irritants.

Competitive success in games is discouraged, but the pre-patients are shifted from group to group according to their abilities. Those with orthopedic problems receive special physiotherapy, therapeutic exercises, massage, and the like. Cold-water showers and steam baths are used extensively. Diets are generally low in animal-fat content.

Ohlstadt handles 125 patients at one time and has a staff of four doctors, several exercise instructors, three nurses, and ten administrative personnel. Sports clothing, bathrobes, and other items of equipment are supplied free.

Obviously Ohlstadt does not promise a complete "cure" for each patient, but the program generally breaks the vicious circle of fatigue, tension, and loss of self-confidence, and it most certainly promotes the understanding for the need of healthy living habits. Each patient receives instructions for a home exercise program and, if necessary, psychological advice is given to maintain the benefits of the program beyond the training period.

Humanitarian values aside, think of what similar centers, or even a pilot center, could do for the individual, for industry, and for labor in this country. A few years ago the United States government appropriated almost $400 million for medical research. But because of a lack of facilities, personnel, and programs, $25 million went begging. Think of what that sum could have done for establishing a reconditioning center. As of now, fantastic sums are needlessly lost on absenteeism, medical care, and hospitalization.

Besides the humanitarian and economic values any American reconditioning center would have, a center would also open up new avenues of research in medicine, areas in which research is absolutely vital. In 1964 Dr. Wilhelm Raab of the University of Vermont College of Medicine held the First International Conference on Preventive Cardiology. Physicians and researchers from all over the world presented papers on exercise and heart disease. It was a magnificent gathering, yet Dr. Raab had to scrimp, scrounge, and beg funds to hold the conference. Many valuable papers were presented.

Dr. Herman K. Hellerstein of Western Reserve University reported on reconditioning programs he had started for heart patients in Cleveland. Among other things, Dr. Hellerstein discovered that recovered heart patients, who still had from 50 to 75 per cent of their coronary artery flow shut off, could be restored to near normal function

178

through exercise. One heart patient, who had suffered a very bad attack, was swimming a quarter of a mile a day.

Dr. M. E. Groover of the University of Oklahoma reported that he had found streaks of dead tissue in the heart muscles of Kenya baboons. Investigation then revealed that the damage had occurred when the baboons were trapped, when they were unable to respond to fight or flight. This condition, Dr. Groover said, may be "related to the mechanisms in the young executive who is caught in an emotional trap and cannot balance his nervous system by physical activity such as running or fighting."

Dr. Daniel Brunner of Tel Aviv reported on investigations of more than ten thousand men and women who were members of Israeli kibbutzim, collective settlements. The settlements were perfect laboratories in that they offered uniform environmental conditions. Each had one common dining room and no differences in living standards. And what did Dr. Brunner find? That heart attacks were two to four times more common among the sedentary kibbutzim workers than they were among the men and women who worked in the fields.

This was just one conference on heart disease and exercise. Think of the progress medicine could make if reconditioning centers and research facilities were established in this country. We could learn a great deal, and what we learned could then be applied to the public at large.

So far little progress has been made in acquainting the public with a real need, the imperative need for physical activity. The President's Council on Physical Fitness, the AMA, the Association for Health, Physical Education and

Recreation have been talking, writing, and arranging meetings to that end. There have been public-relations campaigns, too. But so far the main point has been missed. Physical activity is not a frill that you may indulge in, because it might be helpful and because it might make you more acceptable. **Physical activity is necessary for truly normal living and is an essential factor in disease prevention.** This must be emphasized.

But even when this has been done, we will still have more to do; we must answer the need for exercise. To do this best, we need a national organization, a national foundation, to supervise a country-wide program. Such a foundation would not be without precedent. Pehr Henrik Ling (see p. 34) organized the Royal Swedish Institute for Gymnastics in 1770. This institute has helped Sweden to become a leader in the development of physical training. Then again, it is not new in the United States to have a foundation to further national programs in health. There is the National Foundation for Infantile Paralysis, which has had tremendous success. Before the discovery of the polio vaccine the foundation organized state and local chapters and trained members in exercise therapy for polio victims. The foundation introduced Sister Kenny's system of exercise and treatment, and although a number of physicians were opposed to this at the start, the system was widely taught and provided an excellent basis for the treatment of polio patients.

I would now hope to see a similar foundation for exercise created in this country. The honorary chairman should be the President, as was the case with the foundation for infantile paralysis. This new foundation could establish an institute in which exercise would be the basic subject. This institute could call on all available talents, here and abroad; it might well establish student and teacher exchanges with the Scandinavian countries or others that are advanced in the field. This central institute could set up chapters in every state of the Union. These chapters, in turn, could cooperate with schools, hospitals, private groups, and any established reconditioning centers. The national foundation would have liaison with medical schools and departments of physical education. Within the foundation itself there would be departments to work on such diverse but important factors as liability laws, building codes, city school planning, home planning, city planning and, *of course,* outdoor recreation. The late President Kennedy was very aware of the fact that the President's Council on Physical Fitness did not and could not go much beyond public-relations efforts. He was deeply interested in doing more, and shortly before his death a proposal for just such a national foundation was submitted to him. It is one of our losses that he did not have the time to act on it.

A new approach is essential. As of now, we are not doing the job.

Conclusion

WE HAVE DISCUSSED many things: the effect of our underexercised and stressful way of life on our health, how to determine whether or not we are underexercised and overstressed, and ways to contend with the problem. Intertwined with this physical and emotional problem is an unfulfilled spiritual need.

We have become far removed from the basic things. Our bread comes processed, pre-sliced and packaged; pavements separate us from the earth; cars and planes give us exaggerated ideas of our power and ability to overcome space and time. Often our work is only a small part of a great organized effort, and laboring among the many, we are deprived of the satisfaction of individual personal accomplishment.

We are shielded from the powers of nature—rain, storm, cold, heat—and it takes floods and earthquakes to remind us of the humble place we occupy on this planet.

As we become more sheltered, we become all the more removed from the very forces that have formed and made us.

Since everything is so far removed, we rarely feel prompted to work on ourselves or our own improvement.

Conclusion

We expect others and "things" to do for us what ultimately remains our very own responsibility.

Understanding our sickness and our weakness, and combating them by personal effort—by *doing*—may help reopen old avenues that we have forgotten in the rush of time.

Bibliography

BARZUN, JACQUES, *House of Intellect*. New York, Harper & Row, 1959.

BOYLE, ROBERT, "Report That Shocked the President." *Sports Illustrated,* August 15, 1955.

CANNON, WALTER B., *The Wisdom of the Body*. New York, W. W. Norton & Company, Inc., 1932.

EASTMAN, MAX, "Let's Close the Muscle Gap." *Reader's Digest,* November 1961.

GASTON, SAWNIE, AND SCHLESINGER, EDWARD B., "Injuries to the Low-Back Mechanism." *Trauma*, Philadelphia, London, Harrison L. McLaughlin, W. B. Saunders Company, 1959.

JACOBSON, EDMUND, *Tension Control for Businessmen*. New York, Toronto, London, McGraw Hill, Inc., 1963.

JOLLIFFE, NORMAN, *Reduce and Stay Reduced on the Prudent Diet*. New York, Simon and Schuster, Inc., 1964.

KENNEDY, JOHN F., "The Soft American." *Sports Illustrated,* December 26, 1960.

KRAUS, HANS, *Principles and Practice of Therapeutic Exercises*. Springfield, Charles C Thomas, 1956.

KRAUS, HANS, AND RAAB, WILHELM, *Hypokinetic Disease*. Springfield, Charles C Thomas, 1961.

SELYE, HANS, *The Stress of Life*. New York, McGraw-Hill, Inc., 1956.

STEINHAUS, ARTHUR H., *How to Keep Fit and Like It*. Chicago, The Dartnell Corporation, 1957.

STIMSON, B., "The Low-Back Problem." *Psychosomatic Medicine* G:210, May–June, 1947.

Acknowledgments

I am greatly indebted to Mr. Robert Boyle, who is largely responsible for the final form of this book, and to my wife, Frances Madi Kraus, for making the drawings and diagrams and for helping with the reading of the proofs.

I am especially grateful to M. Lincoln Schuster for his personal interest and encouragement and to Merrill Pollack for his great cooperation and patience in dealing with this very difficult author.

For reading the manuscript and for giving valuable advice and encouragement, I am greatly indebted to Lloyd Appleton, Ph.D., George Burkley, M.D., George Carden, M.D., Eugene Cohen, M.D., Donald Covalt, M.D., Abraham Franzblau, M.D., Muriel Hart, Ellis Hendrix, P.T., Jack Nelson, M.D., Glen Olds, Ph.D., Mr. and Mrs. Martin Steinberg, Frank Stinchfield, M.D., Sonja Weber, D.Sc.